HAVING A BALL AT THIRTY

HAVING A BALL
AT THIRTY

*How I Got Through Cancer
by Writing a Musical*

by
Tom Willner

HAVING A BALL AT THIRTY
How I Got Through Cancer by Writing a Musical

Manufactured and printed in the United States of America

Published by Coz Branding Press, Atlanta, GA

Cover photography – Louis Leon
Cover design – Coz Branding, LLC

Manuscript page production – Benard Owuondo; Winnie Hulme

For information about special discounts, bulk purchases,
or permissions please contact:

info@cozbranding.com
Coz Branding Press
Atlanta, GA
www.cozbranding.com

ISBN 978-0-9995939-2-9

First printing, 2018

1.   2.   3.

TABLE OF CONTENTS

ABOUT THE AUTHOR

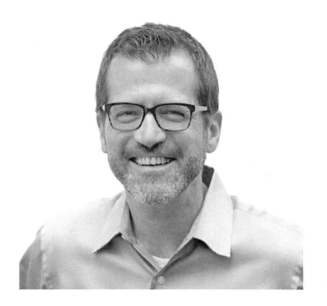

Tom Willner is a longtime resident of Atlanta, Georgia. In addition to a long career in technology, he is an avid musician — composing, playing piano, singing and recording songs when the inspiration strikes. If you catch him at a local venue, you will leave as inspired as you will feel when you finish reading this story. He feels blessed to be a father of three healthy, active, incredible children, and husband to Allyson.

PROLOGUE FROM THE WINGS

By Anne McSweeney

I HAVE LONG BEEN active in medical social work—home health, hospice, dialysis, and the like—as well as working extensively in community relations and community education. About 6 years ago, I started my continuing education company, CEU Creations, for medical professionals (social workers, nurses, case managers and other clinicians) who need ongoing education for licensure.

My motivation in launching the company was actually that many of the continuing education courses and seminars that I have attended were lackluster at best. I knew that when it came to engaging content, I could do better. The "CEU" in *CEU Creations* doesn't stand for "Continuing Education Units" but *"Creative. Educational. Unique."*

Several years ago, I was reading the newspaper and saw Tom Willner's story in the Lifestyle section. I immediately thought how innovative and creative it would be to pair education for healthcare professionals with his musical about the patient experience. Then life happened. Time went on without me looking him up. In mid-2015, fate intervened. I found myself in need of a last-minute replacement presenter for an event where 100 participants had already signed up. So I reached out to Tom with this opportunity and he graciously stepped in. From that first collaboration, there was great synergy between us. It was an amazing seminar experience for everyone; it was indeed *"Creative. Educational. Unique."* That's how we got started together.

The honest, palpable emotional rawness Tom expresses in his story from the patient's point of view is quite unique in the continuing education world. As we plan these training events, we reach out to a number of experts to present. However, we often overlook the valuable viewpoint of the patient's perspective. Pairing the licensed medical professional with a patient in a seminar immediately changes the perspective on the subject matter for the participants. This change of perspective is vital — especially since so many medical centers are committed to providing Patient Centered Care. This is not just a buzzword. There is a continuous push for us all to provide it. If we don't know what the patient's perspective is, how can we provide Patient Centered Care?

My hope for healthcare professionals is that we can help them walk in the shoes of a patient experiencing a traumatic diagnosis, and grasp what that looks like for him/her during diagnosis, treatment, survival, or even end-of-life. What are the biggest issues facing our patients from their point of view? What are the "little things" a patient deals with — the "hurry up and wait" syndrome, the agony of waiting for results, high hopes being dashed — and what can the professional do to improve the experience for the patient? And how can we make them more livable for family members close to the experience?

A few years ago, I had the good fortune of reading a powerful poem (JAMA, 1996) by Stephen Schmidt called "A Piece of My Mind — When You Come Into My Room." Hearing this patient's perspective on how he is so much more than his illness really struck a chord with me. The poem details one patient's life and how it is so important to this patient for his healthcare providers to know the "big picture" about who he really is as a person. A patient is much more than their medical chart. Tom's book echoes this, and as healthcare professionals, if we can gain this understanding early on in our careers, we will be better equipped to serve our patients and their families.

Besides gaining the patient's point of view, another benefit of experiencing Tom's musical is the way it helps us help our patients with coping mechanisms. Tom actually wrote the musical as he was going through cancer treatments. He found this writing to be cathartic. It helped him deal with the pain he was experiencing. If we can pass along creative coping strategies to our patients and their families (and show them the way other patients in their shoes have coped as well), we may be able to shed some light on new ways of coping that might help them to release their own feelings along the way.

Seeing a journey through the patient's eyes helps us as professionals respond by trying, at least, to create a more comfortable, connected experience. This type of insight can be incredibly powerful, especially for physicians who find it challenging when a patient is emotional. In many situations, a physician will respond to a patient's emotions by providing more education about their diagnosis. At these emotional times, patients often need more empathy for who they are as a whole person. They need someone to sit with them and talk to them. And in some cases, they look to their physicians to provide this. As a medical team comes together for a patient, every one of its members must conversationally prepare him for and help him through the roller coaster ride that so frequently accompanies patient care.

Tom's story is not just a cancer story. It's about the whole experience of a scary diagnosis for the patient and his family. And in Tom and Allyson's case, it's also about the risk to a family — a family that may not have formed at all (this will make more sense as you read Tom's story).

Connecting again with Tom's expression of his own patient-centered experience reminds me of my medical social work years, working directly with patients. It so closely parallels what I saw then. I witnessed my patients experiencing many of the emotions that Tom so eloquently describes. A patient is so much more than his/her diagnosis. Tom drives that home. How do we connect with the humanity of the patients and families that we work with? Tom's story reminded me that we need to know more about the patient than just his diagnosis and his numbers. More than the science behind his care. It is my hope that this story can help us get closer to true Patient Centered Care.

Anne McSweeney
*LMSW and President of **CEU Creations**
www.ceucreations.net*

*Tom Willner and Anne's company is **Center Stage Education**. **www.centerstageeducation.com***

THE CAST

Conlan *A cheerful man who feels fortunate as he celebrates his thirtieth birthday. He is happily married to Halle who wants to start a family, but he is enjoying his life and doesn't want to change it. Suddenly, he's diagnosed with cancer and spends the next two years on a physical and emotional roller coaster, battling the disease. His experience and his reactions to his diagnosis are explored by fluctuating between the real and the surreal. He ends up as a father and a changed man with a new perspective on life.*

Halle *Conlan's loving wife who is ready to start a family — even though he is not. After Conlan gets testicular cancer, she puts on a brave face for him, but is privately devastated. At her request, Conlan goes to a fertility clinic during the ordeal in order to ensure they can one day have children. Ultimately, she convinces him to have a child and ends up as a hopeful mother with a new appreciation for life.*

Dr. Saxon *The doctor who helps Conlan fight the cancer through surgery, or the "sword." He is patient and strong. He convinces Conlan to remain hopeful and fight the disease instead of giving up. While Dr. Saxon appears to defeat T.C. in a sword duel, T.C. returns. In a last ditch effort to save Conlan's life, Dr. Saxon sends Conlan to the Wizard.*

T.C. *The personification of Conlan's testicular cancer. She is a smooth, confident character who sees herself as providing an important service to humanity by helping people prioritize* *what's truly important in life. She appears during the surreal segments, intervening where she's not wanted. She battles Dr. Saxon over Conlan in a sword duel, and appears to both harm Conlan and be defeated by Dr. Saxon, but she returns once more.*

Wizard *The oncologist who appears in the surreal segments as a wizard with a magic potion. He is grandiose and confident in himself and the course of action necessary to help Conlan. He states that the way to kill the parasite is to poison the host, and proceeds to administer chemotherapy.*

Three Clown-like Doctors *Part humorous, part frightening, the three clown-like doctors appear in the surreal segments where Conlan deals with the necessary medical tests and procedures.*

All characters can be portrayed with five actors — two women and three men.

OVERTURE

MINOR INCONVENIENCES

I HAD BEEN HAPPILY coasting along towards my 30th birthday with my sweetheart Allyson and our family and friends, enjoying a career going the way I had hoped it would. Life was grand. Until it wasn't anymore.

Scary diagnoses came along to rock my boat. And if that wasn't enough? Several difficult surgeries to get through. Guilt that my earlier reluctance to start a family was doomed to keep us from parenthood. A never-before-experienced fear of death and dying.

Such were the "minor inconveniences" that crashed down on me and turned my good life upside down.

My early denial of the disease and my later acceptance and healing of it led me to pen a full musical — the one I talk about in these pages. My early fears and newfound courage in face of the treatments and procedures that would heal me led me to it. The death of my old perspective and attitudes, and my rebirth out the ashes led to the story captured in the 17 songs of this musical.

I was able to work out my new feelings and emotions by writing songs. I was able to heal (maybe heal better, more completely, if not necessarily faster) as I did what came naturally to me — writing words and melodies to tell a story.

REFOCUSING MY ENERGY

After my diagnosis — which, as you might guess, stirred up a lot of fears, confusion, and other deep and gloomy emotions within me — I started writing in a morning journal. This was inspired by the method described in Julia Cameron's *The Artist's Way*. The journal would be extremely personal, and I wrote whatever I wanted in it. I extensively journaled the ideas for the musical called *Turning Thirty* as they came to me.

I journaled in one notebook after another. In hindsight, this kept my focus positive and creative during a dark, challenging time. I penned the lyrics to each song in my journals, too. I didn't date every one of the songs, but my journal stands as a record of their chronology. It is also a sort of record of how I was dealing (or not dealing) with my changing body and life.

This book describes my journey through the writing of the songs, not in the order they appear in the musical, but in the order they were written.

I am a trained musician, but not a full-time one. Music — especially the *Turning Thirty* musical — is a project for me. I have all my music on my website, ***www.tomwillner. com,*** for those readers who are interested.

I enjoy a number of musical styles, so I used *Turning Thirty* as an excuse to write in a number of styles. I wrote in whatever style seemed appropriate for the lyrics and the emotions. As you know, it is not lyrics alone, but also major and minor keys, beats, and melodies that convey emotions and stories. The musical is not, therefore, composed in a single "classic," "dance," or "Broadway" style of music. It is very much about what was going on for me at the time I penned the song — how I was experiencing my health, my cancer, and my life in general at the time.

COIN TOSS

Every coin has three sides: Heads, it's tragedy. Tails, it's comedy. And then, thank goodness, there's the edge.

My edge, my nudge toward health and back into the happiness that had been shattered by the diagnosis and subsequent medical interventions, was a shift in my perspective. I took charge of the spin I gave events and circumstances. It was all in my mind? Fine. I'd change my mind. I pivoted slightly because that was the best I could do at the time, and my attitude changed. Over time, those course corrections ultimately changed my life.

I find that too few people really believe in free will. Our ability to choose is our free will. I feel impatient now when I hear someone exclaim, "But I had no other choice!" Usually people use this phrase to explain why they have taken some disastrous action. By making a tiny shift in our perspective and attitude, we get to choose something new. Heads or tails. Comedy or tragedy. We do get to choose. In the shock of facing death, I momentarily lost my perspective. I lost my optimism, really quite briefly, though, because I had my wife and my music and so much other help along the way.

I chose to see blessings and happiness in everything. I examined every downer for its hidden positive aspect. I looked for a benefit in every apparent drawback. For every tragic piece of news, I looked for the comic side of things.

I have such a rich life. So much love. An interesting profession that earns me a nice living. I didn't have children when this all began, then I feared I never would. But I am blessed with three of them now—that in itself is a miracle. I decided that I didn't need to see things as heads or tails. My new perspective allows me to choose the edge, to experience adversity not with panic or anger, but with a quiet sort of smile.

As Will Shakespeare said, "*One man in his time plays many parts.*" I took on the role, briefly, of man in despair, screaming, crying, and kicking back. The role of a dying man. I caught myself and gave the coin a spin. That despair is not a role for me. I wasn't cut out for the "Oh, why me, dear Lord?" type of role. It is not a part I want to play. So I don't.

AWAKENING

As I faced my circumstances, I woke up from the pain and distress bit by bit. I stared out the window during the day, and saw people going about their business. Some were nonchalant and looked like they were having a day off. Others raced around and I could feel their tension. I gazed out of the window late into the night, and saw how the moon so gracefully backlit everything spread before my eyes.

Life was moving on out there. Life looked pretty good.

My rational brain had me jump like we all do when we can't figure something out, or don't know some fact. I hopped from website to website, trying to educate myself with real science about what my body was going through. On the other side of that equation, I have always been a creative kind of guy. Music and lyrics, the comedy and the drama of my position came at me at odd times. Left brain, right brain — both still working and doing their jobs for me.

Before a major surgery, the physician agreed to give me an extra week for an overseas trip already planned with my wife. Putting off the life threatening for a celebration of life. I needed — wanted — to celebrate my life every single day. As you will see in the next pages, I sometimes simply did not have the energy to do so. And yet, I bounced back.

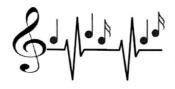

YOUR NUMBER'S UP

"Sometimes you win, sometimes you learn."

~ John C. Maxwell

*"No man is broken because bad things happen to him.
He's broken because he doesn't keep going after
those things happen."*

~ Courtney Milan

*"Bad things can happen, and often do —
but they only take up a few pages of your story;
and anyone can survive a few pages."*

~ James A. Owen, *The Barbizon Diaries: A Meditation
on Will, Purpose, and the Value of Stories*

THINGS HAD BEEN GOING so well for me for so long. 30 years, in fact. I had been very healthy all that time and suddenly, Bam! Here is some cancer. "Cancer?! For Christ's sake, the very same shit that drained the life out of my father! And now it's in me? My number's up. I'm gonna die." Thoughts about my dad flooded in. He had died one short year before of prostate cancer.

Journaling quickly became very personal and intimate as I went through this journey from health to disease and back to health. I'll talk about that as we go along.

Things were actually going pretty well. My wife and I were DINKs — *dual income, no kids.* Both my wife and I travelled a lot for our jobs. Our lives were very Type A — we were always on the go and so we had some unusual ways of getting things done. For example, we put an offer on our house on a Sunday night just prior to both taking trips to different parts of the country. (She went to Maine and I went to California.) During those trips, we heard that the seller had countered through our broker. On our layovers, we accepted the counter proposal via voice mails with our broker, and then we got back on our respective planes as new owners of a house! We still live in it. Our family is still here, growing and thriving in that house. The mundane and exceptional were handled like this when we were apart, pretty smoothly, we thought, and life was good.

Everything was cool. Until it wasn't.

I was at my wife's company retreat. I was one of three husbands out of the hundred spouses that were there. I played tennis and golfed with the spouses while Allyson attended sessions. This was right around my August birthday. It was at the retreat, while showering, that I discovered the lump. I didn't know what it was — ironic, given that I was working at the American Cancer Society. You would've thought that since I had so much information about cancer swirling around me on a daily basis, I would've had a clue. Not! Talk about denial. My wife knew somehow. She had an idea of what it was. She nailed it and made the medical appointment with the urologist.

I think it was August 12, 1999 that I had that appointment, not really thinking about the potential that it could be anything scary at all. The physician never used the word "cancer," but the word "tumor" instead. The doctor said, "It could be a fluid-filled cyst, but we need to biopsy it to see what's what." I'm not sure if I realized at the moment that "biopsy" really meant "remove the whole testicle and figure out if it is cancerous."

I lost my father to prostate cancer the year before. None of what I was hearing said cancer to me. Not the doctor. Not my mind. For me, cancer was for much, much older people, like parents and grandparents. Cancer happened late in life and I wasn't late in my life yet, so it could not possibly be that!

When, one week later and less one testicle, I heard the word cancer, the doctor presented me with two choices:

1. Watch and wait — though what I was waiting for was still really, really murky to me. Or
2. Go for another surgery, after some new scans and tests. It would be for lymph node removal this time, and ensuing biopsy.

Scans showed a couple of lymph nodes that were kind of large. I decided that I was pretty healthy and should just get on with it and get it over with.

CUT IT OUT
The Retroperitoneal Lymph Node Dissection (RPLND) was scheduled for early September. I think it was on September 1. RPLND surgery is pretty aggressive. In fact, looking back, there are no words to describe how aggressive it ultimately felt. I will spare you the gruesome details, but the lymph nodes at issue are in the abdominal area. It involved cutting my torso

open, carefully moving aside the organs there to get to and remove the lymph nodes that are behind them, repositioning my organs again, and closing me up.

BUBBLING UP

The idea for this song, *Your Number's Up*, probably started to germinate on that first day when I sat down with all this new information about not only cancer, but about the reality of cancer inside me. I did what I could to face it and process it. I admit that the processing part only started when I heard the word cancer for the first time during a discussion with my wife. Processing the implications of cancer in my body and my life continued for a long time. Coming to terms with cancer? How does anyone do that?

Even before the RPLND surgery, lots of questions were bubbling up. "Hell, is this what happens when you turn 30?" I wondered. This was a recurring thought, as were many others. "Your number (30) is up, kid." "Thirty years is all I get?" My mind was spinning on and on, over and over, in this vein. It was hard to decipher at first, but I later identified my grief and despair, my anger and bitterness. Why now? Why me?

What could cancer be thinking to be in me like this? My mother-in-law would later call cancer a trickster, but the thought was already lurking in my subconscious. The germ of my personification of cancer was here, in these thoughts.

TAKING FORM

TC, testicular cancer, would sing this song to me. The song would be cancer's words. What would cancer be thinking? Would it be singing a victory tune as it conquered me? Would it be lurking and preying on me and then pouncing?

Moods and melodies went through my head as I wrote this song with cancer as the singer. I would repeat a line of lyrics, and it would take on its own life, formulating its own melody line as syllables and rhymes flowed, coming, going, and finally sticking.

The melodic accompaniment is a strong march that might mark the arrival of an all-powerful invading army. Ominous, haunting, scary, with the final lines repeating themselves. Grim. Ugly.

The melody didn't share that gravitas completely. It was more fluid than that. Combined, the song said, "Here's this person (cancer) or invading force being mean to me. This is how it is and what it does. And I'm its next victim." The cancer was taking form in my mind as a person, a personality, a character. I wanted the lyrics to sound like natural speech from cancer, with a specific meter and a haunting repetition of end line words.

I left the swear words in. I had to give it my real mood.

YOUR NUMBER IS UP

Things have gone so well for you, too well, too well.

Time to cast a spell on you. Time to give you hell.

But what could be the reason for this sudden turn for the worse?

No reason is required if the cause is uninspired. It's just a curse.

Because your number's up. It's time for you to sweat.

Yes, your number's up and thirty's all you get.

That's more than you deserved. I hate to wait so long.

You have so much that is right, so here's some wrong.

Look at you feeling everything is grand.

A little bit of shit can hit you right there where you stand.

When you least suspect it, you won't know what it will be,

*But you'll know it once it's there and you'll be so afraid
to see*

That your number's up. It's time for you to sweat.

Yes, your number's up and thirty's all you get.

That's more than you deserved. I hate to wait so long.

Why should everything be so right,

Why should everything be so right when there is wrong.

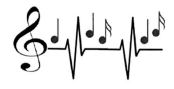

HOW COULD THIS BE

"Am I still attractive? Can I still function?"

~ Tom Willner

"Bitterness is like cancer. It eats upon the host.
But anger is like fire. It burns it all clean."

~ Maya Angelou

"Despair is the price one pays for self-awareness.
Look deeply into life, and you'll always find despair."

~ Irvin D. Yalom

"No, I am not bitter, I am not hateful, and I am not
unforgiving. I just don't like you."

~ C. JoyBell C.

WHO AM I?

O N SOME MORNINGS, JOURNALING was hard. One day I wrote, "I have a lot of thoughts on my mind and I can barely write fast enough." Because of the testicular connection, my mind went to male sexuality and sexual issues. Crap, I wasn't even a father yet! Can I father children? What is my wife's reaction going to be if I can't? Is she going to be repulsed by me from now on? Am I still attractive or is my sex appeal gone forever? Can I still function sexually? Can I even still have sex? I couldn't write fast enough to keep up with the awful, depressing thoughts my mind was spinning out. And my mind seemed to be intent on beating me up pretty hard.

In trying to just write down these basic male sexuality questions, this very masculine aspect of the cancer, I realized I had done absolutely no thinking about any of this before — not ever. I can face it now, years later. But if anyone had asked me to do a stream of consciousness on male sexuality back then, before my diagnosis, I would've had to blow them off. After all, "real men" don't need to deal with anything like that! Ha!

I found myself growing a beard for the first time. My wife has never been too big on beards, and I was happy to avoid growing one. Until I wasn't. Maybe I was compensating for the supposed emasculation of losing a testicle. "A man has a beard," I thought. I wanted my wife to approve of it, too. My mind kept returning to expressions of masculinity and my old (and now changing) assumptions of masculinity.

I hadn't ever felt concerned by men's "emasculation" issues before. Those issues didn't resonate with me. But times and events change perspectives! I definitely felt "less than" after one of my testicles was removed. Thinking back, I can relate to women who've lost a breast. If I'd had a tumor or growth on my thigh, for instance, none of this male drama would have surged up at all. Breasts and balls, though, involve a whole different set of emotions and attachments! Hmm… Maybe I should've written a song about that for the musical.

I also had my own subtler reaction to being emasculated. Wanting more approval and needing to be validated became a new monster for me for a while. My self-confidence evaporated, albeit briefly, and I needed it to come from the outside, which of course never works. On occasion, I just didn't know who I was anymore. My old assumptions about my life were no longer a bedrock of truth on which to base my identity or my future.

RUDE AWAKENING

When we were kids, a childhood friend of mine died of leukemia. My grandmother passed away when I was very young and though cancer was involved, I was unaware of it at the time. I found out later.

In spite of those experiences, I realized I didn't know much about this disease. Those experiences came upon me at an age when I didn't really register any of the implications of disease or understand how my loved ones died. Even when my father died from cancer in his 60s, a year before my own diagnosis, it still felt foreign to me. Then, here I was, at age 30, rebelling against the awareness of my own cancer. I thought that I was far too young to contract it. I was far, far too young to die of it. Cancer is for much older people! How could this be my lot?

I began to wonder if cancer was part of my family's genetics. I found myself much, much more often simply wallowing in the unfairness of it all. My world as I had known it — friendly, fun, loving, secure, and healthy — had turned against me. I despaired that nothing would ever be the same for me again. People would find me "less than" and move away from me. People would imagine that my sense of humor had evaporated (and it had for a while, as I penned out this song).

No one could possibly love the remnants of me that were left after the surgeries and treatments. My world felt insecure and unfriendly. My body had betrayed me and made me lose all that I once held to be real and true.

THE TRIVIALITY OF DRAMA

My definition of "problems" shifted dramatically! My ability to deal with stresses and problems began to expand (and is still expanding today) more and more. I saw petty problems as inconsequential compared to the drama around my cancer.

As I was bitterly cursing the unfairness of this death knell, I still had to watch the people around me getting stressed out by the same old issues as always. They kept on doing their impersonations of drama kings and drama queens. Their complaints and the "terrible" injustices done to them that were still so earth-shattering in their minds started to seem really petty to me at this point. My own drama was bigger than theirs — didn't they know that? "Hey, guys, you don't know what a real problem is," I thought. My fright meter had been turned way up and they were worried about who had again failed to contribute to the lunchroom's coffee kitty — inconsequential nothings in comparison. That sucked. And how could I ever convince them to shut up and hear my tales of pain and fear and despair? I guess I was hurt that their narrow-sightedness prevented them from seeing how much I needed love and attention. I sort of lost my footing around people for a good while. I wasn't used to needing outside comfort, I guess, and there I was seeking it. It was very unsettling.

This song is the reaction to the realizations of 'Your Number's Up', as in "What the fuck? How did this happen? Why me?" I was in grief and despair, anger and bitterness. *Why me?*

I imagined this song early on, interestingly enough, as a dance. It is a 3/4-time waltz. The lead characters (portraying me and my wife) are dancing together and lamenting the circumstances. Cancer dances off to the side. Then the cancer cuts in. When the main character finally notices that cancer has cut in on the dance, his bitterness and anger explode. He is thinking, "What gall you have to mess with me! I don't like you and you have no place cutting in!" I had my song.

HOW COULD THIS BE

Everything was fine. Everything was good.

Now there's only rubble where great buildings once stood.

My life has changed. I've lost my footing, my bearing.

The pages of my life neatly written now are tearing.

How could this be?

I had no reason to believe that this could happen to me.

The world I once knew is no longer true,

And the one that I'm left with is so frightening to see.

How could this be?

Others have their problems. I once had those, too.

Now I'd gladly trade mine for theirs if only that's what I could do.

I used to be so happy. I used to have it made.

Now I feel as though I have a mysterious debt to be repaid.

How could this be?

I had no reason to believe that this could happen to me.

The world I once knew is no longer true,

And the one that I'm left with is so frightening to see,
And the one that I'm left with is so frightening to see.
How could this be?
How dare this be the case! What gall to mess with me!
I've never hurt another, least not intentionally.
What nerve of him to enter my peaceful little town!
He's come into my life and turned it upside down.
I am hurt, I am bitter, and for the life of me
I cannot see how this could be.

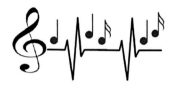

WE WILL FACE THIS FOE

"I focused on the fish."

~ Tom Willner

"A man may learn wisdom even from a foe."

~ Aristophanes

*"When I hear music, I fear no danger.
I am invulnerable. I see no foe. I am related to the
earliest times, and to the latest."*

~ Henry David Thoreau

MORNING JOURNALING

I WAS IN THE days after being diagnosed from the biopsy results and going through the RPLND surgery. As I stated earlier, one of the first things I did for myself and my healing before the September 22 surgery was to start regularly journaling. The journal I kept was my creative outlet and a way to refocus my emotions, but it was also an astonishing stimulus for me to 'brain-dump' a creative stream of consciousness for this musical. It was as though the musical — with all its cathartic messages and music — was right under the surface, just waiting for me to grab a pen and my journal.

It started quite simply. One of my best childhood friends had sent me *The Artist's Way* by Julia Cameron.

I knew that I'd be at home recuperating from major surgery and *The Artist's Way* gave me a way to tap into my creativity. *The Artist's Way* process of journaling was an extra impetus for me to explore this health experience creatively. It allowed me to explore what was going on through this series of procedures and my stages of recovery.

I took a cheap old wide-ruled 70-page notebook purchased at the drugstore and created an entry. I just wrote "Turning Thirty the Musical" at the top of the page. I immediately listed most of the cast of the show. Many of the song titles came to me in that same sitting and I jotted them down one after another on the same page. Every other detail about the musical and the songs flowed from this entry.

The song "We Will Face this Foe" came out during my first attempt on September 22 to do *the Artist's Way* morning journaling. I wrote lyrics for both "How Could This Be?" and "We Will Face this Foe" that same day. I put the lyrics right down in the same old drugstore notebook.

THE SURGERY

The major surgery was successful. It was followed by a hellish, grueling week in the hospital. It was the hardest thing I'd gone through in my life. When I woke up, the pain was crazy harsh. I wasn't surprised at the concept of pain-after-surgery. I was braced for it, or so I imagined. My own actual pain was a big surprise, though. The epidural for the pain didn't take. The anesthesiologist went to morphine. I seem to recall her saying something like, "Screw this. Give him morphine." With morphine, I was really still in pain, but I just didn't care. I was the observer of the pain rather than the one experiencing it. The pain floated behind my drug-induced euphoria.

During my week in the hospital after surgery, I had to relearn how to eat, go to the bathroom, and walk. I got to the point where I was able to hobble around, pee, and poop. The goal was also to be back on solid food (and get off the IV nutrition) before leaving hospital care. Like a baby, I went from purees and Jell-O to solid foods.

That whole week, I had an NG (nasal gastric) tube — really gross — to drain the bile. My body fought it, which is natural, since it is a foreign body. A scab started to form around the tube. The clear plastic container of my bile was actually suspended on the wall. Yuck. The tube was one of the worst aspects of that week. It gave me no end of grief. The tears I shed on the day it was removed were half from pain and half from joy. I was grateful to have the tube out of my body.

I was finally home resting and recovering. At home, my orders were to continue walking as upright as possible in order to build strength, especially in my abdomen. I was ordered to eat well and rest a lot.

I was groggy for most of the hospital stay. Blurry thoughts would float in and out without me being able to really grab them or develop them. There was a white board in my hospital room. My mother-in-law drew a large fish on it as a focal point for me. I focused on that to realize I was present. I still see the board and drawing today in my mind.

CREATIVITY FLOURISHES

But, once home, that grogginess did an about-face and turned into hyper-creativity, with fast thoughts whizzing around in my head. I wrote the *Turning Thirty* concept, characters, and song titles in my journal as I mentioned before. I wrote the titles of six or seven songs almost without lifting the pen, without pondering them or trying to figure anything out. It all just came through me with great ease and clarity. It was like I was a channel or a vessel for the ideas that were being poured into me. I had tapped into something that just flowed through me from the Divine, the Collective Consciousness — whatever you want to call it. It flowed quickly and effortlessly. Many creative people speak of this state of being.

As a composer, I had never written a full play or musical. I'd never had a concept for one before now. Being fed top down for the first time with so much creative content and so many song titles coming to me in a single rush after I wrote the words "Turning Thirty" had never happened for me before. I was literally singing the tunes out to myself and on the piano, in a non-stop session of creativity. I just knew what the song lyrics were going to be about. This was the first time I had ever been given an entire concept and all the detail so easily and all at once.

After "How Could This Be," I wrote "We Will Face This Foe." This is the doctor's song, sung by the doctor character who is inspired by my real urologist. The character represents all my doctors, really, but I focused on one physician for this song.

BACKSTORY

In dealing with cancer, the best doctors (like the ones I had) share with you as much real information as they can, to help you rise out of the emotional side of this devastating news and into becoming a partner with them in your healing. This song really reminds cancer patients of this. Yes, we feel devastated. Life as we knew it is over and life itself may be over. We are deathly afraid. Afraid of death. We would like to choose the option of hiding our heads in the sand. We want everyone to stop trying to cheer us up because our grief and fear are so tangible. Medical science has faced this foe before and has the means at its disposal to fight it. A lot of times, you just don't feel like you can make a quick decision to take the right action. You are so foggy with the grief, fear, and anger that it is hard to accept what is happening. Acceptance of the cancer — accepting that yes, cancer is in your body, it happened to you, and requires attention — is what helps you fight.

THE LYRICS

So I wrote the song lyrics about the doctor, who is cautiously optimistic and encouraging me to fight. My constitution is strong and I can do this, he says. I don't hear him at first. I am floundering in the fear and reluctance to fight. The doctor succeeds in bringing me around to his viewpoint. We join at the end, agreeing to fight the culprit called cancer.

I penned this song about the forces of good (represented by the doctor character) in one sitting. Then I played with the lyrics that had come top-down to me a bit more than for other songs. My thought was that a doctor would represent the forces of good that would help me fight the forces of evil. This was the first time that I was consciously writing a duet from the start.

I was trying to have a conversation in song. The assumption was that we were in the doctor's office. Halfway through the song the main character joins the doctor's soliloquy. The main character bounces off the doctor's lyrics while looking at the audience, and later sings as a call-and-response to the doctor. The doctor is trying to motivate me, his patient, to fight the cancer. Then we come together in voice for the final lyrics.

This song was really rewarding to me — it was the first duet I'd ever written. I liked the call-and-response form it took.

"We Will Face this Foe," where the Doctor is singing, is the flip side of "Your Number's Up," where TC, the cancer, is singing.

This is again a march, with the same melodic theme as "Your Number's Up" — appropriately, perhaps, as it is the opposite of that message. It is the counter-offensive to the previous attack by the cancer. It calls to mind the sort of time when "the people rally," so to speak. The piece is in a minor key.

I like that I have the same melodic theme in both this and "Your Number's Up" as they really are the two sides to one coin. This melody is not the exact same all the way through as "Your Number's Up" — a brand-new melodic section comes in for the back-and-forth between the singers — but it leads back to the same melody in the chorus.

I identify for you the characters singing to make the lyrics of the song clearer.

WE WILL FACE THIS FOE

DR. SAXON:

Look at you feeling sorry for yourself.

Pull yourself together. Get your will down off the shelf.

I've battled him before. I can help you do what's right.

I don't know if we'll win, but I do know we can fight.

Together on this journey we must go
For together we will face this foe.
Sometimes you may fall and you may even die.
Though you may not defeat him you must try.
You have the means at your disposal to beat him. There's no trick.
Set aside your fear for to win we must be quick.
Don't let him hurt your will. Stand firm. Listen to me.
Summon all your strength. Be prepared and you will see
That together on this journey we must go,
For together we will face this foe.
Sometimes you may fall and you may even die.
Though you may not defeat him,
Though you may not defeat him you must try.

CONLAN:
I never asked for this.
I don't want to play this game.
I wish it would just go away
As quickly as it came,
But maybe there is hope
In something he has seen.
Yes, maybe he can help me
And show me what he means.

DR. SAXON:

He's a crafty little bastard.

CONLAN:

I never asked for this.

DR. SAXON:

He'll attack when you are down.

CONLAN:

I don't want to play this game.

DR. SAXON:

He'll hide 'til you forget him.

CONLAN:

I wish it would just go away.

DR. SAXON:

Then he's sure to come around.

CONLAN:

As quickly as it came.

DR. SAXON:

But he's not without a weakness.

CONLAN:

But maybe there is hope.

DR. SAXON:

He works like a machine.

CONLAN:

In something he has seen.

DR. SAXON:

I tell you I can help you.

CONLAN:

Yes, maybe you can help me.

DR. SAXON:

Let me show you what I mean.

CONLAN:

Yes, show me what you mean.

DR. SAXON and CONLAN:

That together on this journey we must go,
For together we will face this foe.

DR. SAXON:

Sometimes you may fall.

CONLAN:

And I may even die.

DR. SAXON:

Though you may not defeat him.

DR. SAXON and CONLAN:

Though you may not defeat him, we must try.

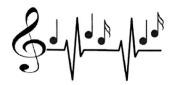

GET THROUGH THIS
WITH YOU

"Will she stay with me through this?"

~ Tom Willner

*"Be strong, be fearless, be beautiful.
And believe that anything is possible when you have
the right people there to support you."*

~ Misty Copeland

*"Therefore encourage one another and
build one another up, just as you are doing."*

~ 1 Thessalonians 5:11

A WEEK AFTER THE RPLND surgery, I left the hospital for more rest and recovery at home. I had a lot of time to think and journal.

As I said, I wrote anything I liked in my notebook. I journaled about my irregular bowel movements after surgery as my "lousy shits." The male sexuality issues came back to mind. I often wrote about or to my wife Allyson in the journal.

FLASHBACKS

I was thinking about my dad and wrote, "I'm planning to go see dad today." The pictures and memories around my parents' house reminded me how much I missed him. Of course, he had passed away the year before. I had regrets about missing dad on occasions when I could've gone to visit, or had been traveling and didn't get out to see him. There were especially the 3 or 4 times my brother urged me to come visit because he thought "this is it" for dad. I wrote, "I hope I can be half the dad you were." I realized I was journaling this entry about my dad one year after his death — to the day.

I'd been sleeping poorly and having lots of dreams. My journal was right there to capture my dream thoughts or stories.

The title of this song refers to Allyson and me getting through this health crisis of mine. I think she contributed, albeit unknowingly, to the song. For the first time in a song, I was trying to speak on her behalf in her half of the lyrics. I projected — based, of course, on having literally gone through this with her — what I thought was going on in her head.

The lyrics came fairly spontaneously. I didn't have to rewrite them much. The lyrics are rife with uncertainty about what was going to happen — and with fear and worry on my part about whether she would be here for me, stay with me through this. Would she be there to catch me if I fell? I'd never expected to be in this type of circumstance anytime in my life. I was fearful about not knowing how this was all going to end. She sings the same lines of worry and wonder as I do. We seem to be reading each other's minds and feeling the same concerns. Love has the final word as far as an expressed emotion — we are there for each other.

It is a duet, a ballad, a love song between two people in love dealing with something very difficult — which is exactly what our situation was. We were two people who had loved each other for a long time, facing our first real shared crisis.

I took this song concept as an opportunity to let the lyrics define the musical and melodic style. I wanted to remain really open to what the lyrics would direct. The song starts in 3/4-time, though it is not really a waltz. The first two verses are an exchange about shared fear. I change then to a 4/4-time signature, also changing to a new tempo and key, with the duo singing in harmony — perhaps to represent that my whole life is changing. The singers are affirming that they're feeling the very same things, expressed in the same lines. I move back into 3/4 time as the lyrics conclude.

Later, after a stage show, that 3/4 time ending changed. It turned out that since this song ends Act One, it needed a different closing flourish. The stage version remains in 4/4 time to the end and other actors (the doctor and cancer) come in for a final chord of voices.

The call to fight the cancer, the affirmation of love and support all mesh together in a hopeful finish, as everyone sings, "I'll be here" — telling me that we'll get through this journey together. We are letting love conquer all fears and concerns. Loving support has the final word. I had my song.

Here are the lyrics. I give you the character voicing the lyrics to allow you to see the call-and-return.

GET THROUGH THIS WITH YOU

CONLAN:

I don't know what's happening to me.

I don't know what the end of this will be.

Hold me now. I'm so afraid. I can't see straight at all.

Will you be there to catch me if I fall?

HALLE:

I don't know why this had to be.

I don't know what the end of this will be.

What will we do? I'm frightened too. I don't know what to say,

But I'll be here every moment, every night, and every day.

CONLAN and HALLE:

Well, I never had expected to be where we are today,

And it frightens me to think about the price that we might pay.

I don't have answers, but I know the only thing to do.

I'll be here to get through this with you.

HALLE:

You're the one I rest my head upon when I go to bed.

CONLAN:

You're the one who calms the demons running round inside my head.

HALLE:

You're the one I long for when I am alone.

CONLAN:

You're the one who showed me love like I've never known.

CONLAN and HALLE:

Well, I never had expected to be where we are today
And it frightens me to think about the price that we might pay.
This must be so hard for you and it's hard for me too.
I'll be here to get through this with you.

HALLE:

I'll be here.

COMPANY:

Together, on this journey we must go.

CONLAN:

I'll be here.

COMPANY:

For together, we will face this foe.

HALLE:
Right here.

COMPANY:
Sometimes you may fall and you might even die.

CONLAN:
Right here.

COMPANY:
Though you may not defeat him.

CONLAN and HALLE:
I'll be here to get through this.

COMPANY:
We must try, must try.

CONLAN and HALLE:
With you, with you.

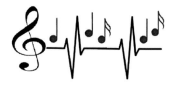

I'M HERE FOR YOU

"They are angels. I was blessed."

~ Tom Willner

*"It is impossible to see the angel unless you
first have a notion of it."*

~ James Hillman

"A nurse... is an angel with a stethoscope."

~ Terri Guillemets

I WAS WARNED THAT it would take my body about 3 months to fully heal and recover from my major surgery in September. On October 15, I was back in the waiting room at my urologist's clinic — back to the place it all started — to see my urologist post-surgery. I was functional again, but still having some pain and discomfort in my remaining testicle. I was hoping it was just a normal part of dealing with post-surgery. There was the underlying worry that it wasn't.

Allyson's brother's first child was born on the 15th, so there were a number of family members in town. It was a happy event, but at this stage of my recovery, still a bit tiring for me.

Allyson got pregnant before my RPLND, the natural way. We'd thrown caution to the wind and decided we could make it happen. As it happily turned out, we found out she was pregnant the very same day we discovered we'd no longer be able to have children the natural way...

I missed a day journaling on October 21. The day before, Allyson and I lost the baby she was carrying.

The bad news just didn't seem to end. I'm feeling a little tired of all the shit, shit, shit. I'm bitter and I'm hurt.

So much life going on all around me — and not all of it happy. I'm not doing well emotionally — my inner child got really bitchy and sad, I have to admit. I'm sad and I don't want to be a sad adult. My soul is injured — when emotional and physical pain keep on coming at me like this, the soul takes a hit. The mind takes a hit.

DREAMS AGAIN

During this period, in addition to having dreams about masculinity, I started having dreams about work. Obviously it was bugging me and I felt some kind of self-inflicted pressure to go back to work. There was a major reorganization going on at work, and it really seemed like a little bit too much for me. I found myself starting to question my life and career decisions. I had lots of lucid dreams throughout this recovery period. I was only about 75% back. I dreamed about feeling stranded, as if everyone else was pressing on without me. I wanted to be back 100%, yet I wondered if I would be, in life and at work. This was, I think, a lot about my impatience with the long, slow process and the amount of time recovery was taking.

I'd had thoughts about writing some dialog for the musical, but I kept coming back to my dreams. My conscious thoughts were focused on getting back to work and my routine. On October 4, I indeed got back to work, albeit from home for four or five days.

All of this bad news, self-administered pressure to get back into the swing of life, and the strain of trying to heal my body amidst it all underlies this song.

THE SONG

I listened to the five prior songs I had penned and my reaction was, "They're pretty fucking awesome." I was still very inspired by "How Could This Be," and in particular "Get Through This with You." I felt it was one of the best things I'd ever written up to that point.

I wrote the song "I'm Here for You" a couple of months later than those prior ones. I'd finished up my original notebook and started another one like it. I'd started to audio record some of the songs myself, with piano and my voice.

As for the concept of the song, Allyson's step-grandmother Diana came to see me in the hospital during the RPLND recovery week. She had worked in some capacity in a hospice and she was amazing to me. Incredibly nice. Ridiculously sweet. Why? Because that's who she was! She was really so very kind. She spent more time with me than anyone. She'd walk and sit with me. She was an endless source of helpfulness during that week. She is thus largely the impetus for this song — as well as, of course, the other women around me, especially Allyson and her mother.

The song is inspired by Diana, but I truly included all the women, family members and nurses, involved in my care. I was truly blessed with the gift of their combined care at that time. I believe oncology nurses are as close to real-life Angels as we can possibly get. It's hard work on all fronts. I later found out these nurses experience high job turnover. This is my homage to them all.

I often start writing a lyric, opening myself to think of melodies as the words start flowing. I can put music to words more easily than the opposite. The words and what they convey is almost always first. I didn't fall this time into my usual rut of forcing the music to the lyric right away — I focused on the words first.

This is also a duet, interestingly. I say this because the two characters both sing, but not to each other. It's not really a conversation. It's as if each one is explaining their own perspective of the story.

It is in a major key, yet in a slower ballad style. I intended it to be sweet, like the people it was about. Some of the words are derived from my continuous gratitude and awe that these women know exactly what to say and what to do. She — whichever she it may be — takes care of me.

I'M HERE FOR YOU

(all lines marked 'Halle' are shared among all my angels)

HALLE

I know you're hurting. I can ease your pain.

I know you're frightened. I can keep you sane.
Your battle's almost over. It's time for you to rest.
Though you may feel cursed, realize you're blessed.

CONLAN

She knows exactly what to say, what to do.
She's an angel.

HALLE

I'm here for you.

CONLAN

She gets me what I need, lets me do what I should do.
She takes care of me.

HALLE

I'm here for you.

CONLAN

Who is this person? Why is she so good to me?
She helps me to heal. She compels me to see.

HALLE

I know where I am needed: here right next to you.
I can comfort you and help you heal, and that is what I'll do.

CONLAN

She knows exactly what to say, what to do.
She's an angel.

HALLE

I'm here for you.

CONLAN

She gets me what I need, lets me do what I should do.
She takes care of me.

HALLE

I'm here for you.

HALLE

You may feel isolated, but you are not alone.
If you need strength, I have some to give.
Think of where you want to be, then take that first step,
To bounce back you must stand, you must walk. You will live.

CONLAN

She knows exactly what to say, what to do.
She's an angel.

HALLE

I'm here for you.

CONLAN

She gets me what I need, lets me do what I should do.
She takes care of me.

HALLE

I'm here for you.

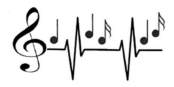

THE BEST JOB IN THE WORLD

"Is that all there is?"

~ Tom Willner

"The mystery of human existence lies not in just staying alive, but in finding something to live for."

~ Fyodor Dostoyevsky, *The Brothers Karamazov*

ALLYSON WAS CONSULTING IN the medical industry at this time and would be off on travel, usually four days at a time. I happily journaled every time she would arrive back home.

I'm starting to slowly get back into music. My friend Ben, with whom I played shows, asked if I was up for a December gig at *Eddie's Attic,* and we scheduled that.

I wrote a lyric called "I'm Not Myself," but never did the music for it. It did not find its way into the musical.

I grew the big beard — a big Grizzly Adams beard, with neck hair and all. I just let it go for a while. But pretty quickly after seeing a picture of myself with the beard, I asked myself, "What was I thinking?!" Allyson didn't like it, so I trimmed it very short.

In mid-November, I was at last on my first business trip after surgery, travelling first class and sitting next to a friendly man. I didn't journal much about my health, really, but I had a bad cough that wouldn't seem to go away.

GOING WITHIN

At this point, I'm really starting to think about what I should be doing with my life. Back at work, I wondered, "Is that it? Is that all there is? This incredibly frightening thing happened to me and I just kind of pick up where I left off?"

I asked myself what to do for my inner child, which had been put through such turmoil over the past several months — and "work on the musical" came to mind. I definitely needed a couple of happy, funny, light, humorous songs. This wasn't one of those, but that was the direction my mind was going at the time.

"Have a ball" and "best job in the world" were the exact words that I journaled. I thought about TC (Testicular Cancer) as a singer for some songs, with a lyric about how much fun it is for him to mess with other people's lives. I could imagine him singing about his fame, notoriety, and power, his hobnobbing with the rich and famous, and everyone else, too, as he puts them through what I went through. He believes he brings out the best in people and reminds them of what is important. "No," I thought. "It doesn't have to be grim, even if cancer was the singer — it could be dark-funny."

My mother-in-law introduced me to the literary concept of the trickster who is smart and sees himself as a good guy contrary to our own terrified view of him. He perhaps has some secret knowledge that he uses to play tricks, to disobey rules with impunity, and to disrupt normal life so it will re-establish itself in a new way. I began to see TC as a trickster like this. That led me to these words: "Once I'm inside your family, it's easy for me to visit your children." Not wanting that terrifying image in any listener's head, I left it out of the song.

I had been journaling extensively about reexamining my values and what was important to me. As I penned my thoughts in my journal, TC was really saying what was going on in my life and my head just then. I wrote, "Holy cow, that just flowed out of me. It's time to write the next song!"

This character — TC, testicular cancer — presented himself in such a different way than anyone would imagine. So I made it jazzy, but in minor key. The material is still kind of dark. It is, after all, cancer who is singing.

I wrote it for a splashy showman on stage, with a long coat and tails and a top hat. That sort of image seemed right. TC indeed displays a bit of arrogance at his fame, power, and notoriety. He is indiscriminate in that he can and does mess with anyone in really scary ways, yet acts like he's helping them out. I imagined the various ways TC is able to get to anyone. He partners with things people enjoy doing, like smoking and lying for hours in the sun on the beach. Because of TC, we get to feel noble as we make charitable contributions to cancer research and lobby the government for more environmental anti-pollution controls.

As it turned out, I cast a woman as TC in the stage production, although until then I had always heard TC speaking to me as a male character. In this male-dominated society, we always start with a premise that if there is an aggressor, it is a male. A threat to my masculinity from this female TC — why not? From a production standpoint, this also worked to balance the cast, since the doctors and other cast were male. This also played well for "Masturbating in a Cup," as you will see later.

I have written the lyrics as universal, but at the song's end, I understand it very personally. TC is there, reminding me that I have been questioning my life's purpose and the value of various things in my life — my values, period. TC says that he is what makes life worth living — not a stupid job, or all that worthless crap you get caught up in. Without me, says TC, you wouldn't know what to do.

The music builds to a final, more flamboyant verse. TC sings the entire song.

THE BEST JOB IN THE WORLD

I have fame and fortune and notoriety.

I hobnob with the rich and famous, the dregs, and everyone in between.

People think I am awful, but I don't see it that way.

I bring out the best and worst in everyone, regardless of what they say.

Now I can make the powerful weak

And I can make the very rich poor.

Unite the masses against me.

Yes, that is what I'm for.
You see, I got the best job in the world.

I got the best job in the world.
I got the best job in the world.
I got the best job.

Would you like to sign up for my service? There are so many
ways to participate.
I partner up with all the things you love. If you don't want me
around, don't take the bait.
Would you care for a smoke? How about a day at the beach
out in the sun?
Take the new gas guzzler out for a spin, now wouldn't that
be fun?
Try some chemicals to help your food grow,
And other great products you can't do without.
The leftover stuff in your water and soil
Is nothing to get too concerned about.

I got the best job in the world.
I got the best job in the world.
I got the best job in the world.
I got the best job.

Hold on, now I take from insurance companies. No one likes
them anyway.

I give to the medical industry. Not a bad deal, I would say.

What about science and research? They need a good riddle or two.

If they already had all of the answers, what would be left for them to do?

See, I'm not so bad. In fact, you need someone like me.

I help to make your life worth living,

Not your stupid jobs or your worthless stuff and all that shit that nobody's giving.

I bring purpose. I return focus. You'll reexamine values, what's important to you.

You hate me because I cause pain, but without me you wouldn't know what to do.

I got the best job in the world.

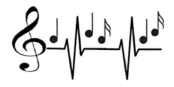

HURRY UP AND WAIT

"Speed has never killed anyone. Suddenly becoming stationary, that's what gets you."

~ Jeremy Clarkson

"Some people, surely, die on the way to something. Then we call them the late so-and-so."

~ Maira Kalman, from *Hurry Up and Wait*

"Nature does not hurry, yet everything is accomplished."

~ Lao Tzu

NORMAL LIFE WAS CREEPING back in and I found myself struggling with that. I felt I was struggling with the same old things that were in my life before this diagnosis. I was struggling especially with day-to-day work and its related travel. I had a few house projects going on, one with our porch — a creative outlet, of the do-it-myself type. Ironically, given what I'd been through, I didn't feel like I was treating myself in a very healthy way. The usual culprits of too much food and not enough exercise or restful sleep were to blame.

At the end of the RPLND, my doctor had told me they found no evidence that the cancer had spread. I thought it was over — I was jubilant! I imagined that I just had to recover, so I beat myself up a bit about not paying better attention to having a healthy lifestyle. By December, though, I was largely healed up from the September surgery, as predicted. I felt well enough to travel to New Jersey for the holidays to visit family and some people I hadn't seen in a long time.

Between September and December, I discovered that I had a potential side effect from the surgery known as *retrograde ejaculation* (the entry of semen into the bladder, from which it is recoverable, instead of going out through the urethra during ejaculation). This was yet another part of the emotional roller coaster ride that we were on.

In December 1999, however, I found out that I did not have retrograde ejaculation as I had supposed. Instead, I had a complete lack of emission of sperm — meaning that eventually I would not produce any sperm at all. What I'd deposited in the sperm bank, prior to my September surgery, would more than likely be all the sperm I'd ever have. Allyson and I were going to the fertility clinic, feeling it was time after our respective recoveries to look at an in-vitro fertilization (IVF) solution.

PERHAPS A MUSICAL

I was starting to toy with more than just penning songs. I began the stage production book for my musical, *Turning Thirty*. I took another shot at "Life is Good" and failed again to get it just right. As I wrote some dialog for a few scenes, I came up with the concepts for two more songs including this one, "Hurry Up and Wait," about checking in with doctors for tests and spending more time in waiting rooms than anywhere else. The other concept I came up with then was the one for "Masturbating in a Cup," a song about the hilarity and humor of going to a sperm bank.

"Hurry Up and Wait" just flowed. My pen hurried through the lyrics, which poured out easily and all at once. I simply put the title at the top of my journal page and just kept writing the words until it was complete. Clearly, I already had melodies in mind as I penned the words, including a counterpoint line by a pair of backup singers. I literally, at the bottom of the page, penned in the letters DFDCFCEF — the actual notes for the counterpoint the backups would be singing. It was my shorthand way of scoring the song.

A good friend of mine grew up in acting and theater, and he'd sent me a tape of songs in musicals. "Hurry Up and Wait" sounds, to me at least, like a traditional or standard Broadway musical number. Not rock, a march, or a waltz. The melody and time signature instead bring the vibe of a clock ticking — something that brings urgency to the lyrics. It's in 2/4-time, but not with standard beats. Each line has 14 beats with seven two-beat measures. Not usual, but I bent the music to fit what I wanted to say.

Interestingly, playing with the tempo and time signature are about communicating urgency and rushing about — time. The words are also naturally about time. It is all based on the ticking of a clock. It's all communicating how we have to go fast to complete something, then fall back from the pace to sit and wait around. Like hurrying to get to an appointment on time, then finding out your person is far behind schedule and asks you to sit and wait.

The doctors and nurses are being playful, manipulating me sort of like I'm their marionette. It's the doctor singing the main song, with nurses singing backup. They are very matter of fact: "Sir, you've gotta do this test, take that sample, go here, gotta figure out what's wrong, go there, then come back. Queue up. Wait." Then the song comes back to the main character, frustrated and angry at this pace and process. He is lamenting how very much he hates this hurry-up-and-wait.

HURRY UP AND WAIT

3 DOCTORS TAKE TURNS SINGING ONE LINE

Gotta get a test.

Gotta do what's best.

Gotta figure out what's wrong.

Just a little prick.

Don't worry. It'll be so quick.

No, it won't take very long.

There's only one way to be sure.

We have to take a look.

Gotta stick to the procedure.

Gotta do it by the book.

Take a little bit from here.

Drain a little bit from there.

Send it off to analyze it.

Quickly now, don't jeopardize.

ALL

The chance we have to tell what's going on.

3 DOCTORS TAKE TURNS SINGING ONE LINE

Gotta get a test.

Gotta do what's best.

Gotta figure out what's wrong.

Gotta figure out what's wrong.

Just a little prick.

Don't worry, it'll be so quick.

No, it won't take very long,

Not very long.

[DOCTOR 2 & 3 begin "bah" vocals, one taking low, one taking high]

DOCTOR 1

There's only one way to be sure. We have to take a look.

Gotta stick to the procedure. Gotta do it by the book.

Take a little bit from here. Drain a little bit from there.

Send it off to analyze it. Quickly now, don't jeopardize

The chance we have to tell what's going on.

DOCTOR 2 & 3

And when that part of you gets to the queue

At one of the few places that do

What we all knew we had to do
To figure out what's up with you,
You have to wait.

CONLAN
I can't take this! I gotta know right now.
The waiting just might kill me. No, I do not know how
I'll be able to stand watching every grain of sand
Slowly tick away the time. This should be a crime,
To make us sit and fret about the results that we might get.
Oh, how so much I hate to hurry up and wait.

JOURNAL

There have been an extraordinary amount of things happening to me that has affected my sexuality as of late. Perhaps its my embarrassment dealing with it all. Perhaps questions like - Am I still attractive? Can I still function?

Another thing on my mind is this whole beard thing. I'm not sure why it's important to me. I want to have a beard, but I also want Alyson & others to think it looks good. I'm not sure what's up with the whole acceptance thing. Perhaps I should not care what others think. It is, after all, something I'm doing only for myself.

I also think that the whole creativity thing is very important to me too. I really want to write the music to this musical. The first song poured out of me pretty quickly - I'm still trying to find the others. I think the story is a good one, it's something I want to do. I had a dream that is still very strong in my head about one of the creatures of Goth Park. I met him and we let it sit and he wanted to spend the time on his trip with me. But I was going to NJ to see mom and it was sad, though I really wanted to stay. There seems to

September 22, 1999

the whole story of my past 2 months down so I can use it as the premise of my musical as well as an easy cut and paste for my emails.

I am planning to go see dad today. The pictures around the house are all happy/sad reminders of the most incredible guy in my life. Good god do I miss him. I think maybe some of the hurt is still that I missed seeing him that last time by a few hours. Dad please forgive me - I was on my way. I'm so sorry I didn't get to see you one last time on the day I was coming. One year ago today. I hope I can be half the dad you were. My little one will be a tribute to you, dad. I know you really loved your dad too. I'm going to do my best to make sure I stay healthy, 'cause I know the Shifner dads don't have the best track records. Hopefully I won't have to battle cancer ever again, but if I do, or I have to battle some other disease or ailment, I'll be strong. I hated this experience, and while I'd do my best to avoid it in the future, that will be through being healthy not avoiding doctors.

September 24, 1999

It's 6:45 am and I just woke from the most horrible nightmare. I was freaked out before I went to bed about my testicle hurting and thinking that it too has a tumor now. The dream was about this family and this house. The "father" was this older man, thin, with gray-white hair. He kind of "ran"

10-10-99

October 10, 1999

Well it's 11:00 and here I sit in the waiting room at Emory Clinic to see Dr. Issa. The place it all started. I'm a little nervous about my visit because of my ball. I only have one, and I don't want it to be problematic too. I hope he says it's normal, or otherwise eases my mind somehow. I have so much to talk to him about it's kind of weird. I wish Allyson were here with me.
        I worked on the musical last night. I

October 15, 1999

a child together, too. But the difference I think is if we weren't able to, I'd be ok, but I'm not so sure she could handle it. It scares me a lot, 'cause I've never seen her be quite so disturbed and have anything only her as weak + depressed as this. Last night's "date" was helpful I think. It was good for me - the first sort of spending/release in a while.
    My soul is injured. When something pounds away at you both mentally + physically it eventually starts hurting you spiritually. That's what all of this has done to me. Ali's mom said something yesterday that she is angry with God. That is pretty major for her, seeing as how she is quite the religious person. I suspect something but I no longer recall.
    God I'll be so happy when my ball is better. It does seem better. It looks better, I believe it looks/feels better but I'm so reluctant to believe that because it's still tender & just want it to feel normal again. Not that I'll ever feel normal

September 25, 1999

Wow life is quite strange these days. All sorts of talk about IVF and my testicles still hurting. I do get to go masturbate again at the clinic. The ol' weird experience, but this time I pee in a cup and they see about getting sperm from my pee. Weird wacky shit. So I played my songs for Cris and Allyson and decided that my Guyphys Girl is not cool. I will most likely trash that song. I did get a cool response from the others, however, so that's good. Allison cried out "Get Through This With You."

November 6, 1999

sit on me. I can't deal with it all. What can I do? My life is too hectic and I need some time to myself. Everyone keeps pulling in all directions and I just want to scream NO! STOP IT! Damn this is my life! AAAARRGH!! What the hell am I supposed to do? I can't get a grip. I can't seem to shake this feeling feeling. I must go to a shrink. What is up with me? How can I shake this?! I'm not healthy. Shit!! I am so angry, bitter and grumpy.
    11-15-99

November 14, 1999

to write that is. To write helps me figure out
what's wrong with me. This particular cracker
is very tasty. I miss my family. I think
that that wasn't a cracker but a biscuit. And
it's damn gouda. (Can you guess what kind of
cheese I'm eating? The two work very well
together.
  So what would I do today if there were
no boundaries? First I'd go to some place where
there's a huge body of water — ocean, lake, whatever
but BIG. And I'd go for a walk. Breathe in the
fresh air. Sip on some fruit juice or juice of some
kind — very fresh. I'd grab a bite to eat in
Paris at a street vendor — some bread. I'd sit
at a gorgeous grand piano and play + sing for a
long time. I'd have several friends or a couple
like Jo & or S & D or T & S, etc. over to play some
games + chat. I'd laugh + laugh. We all
would. I'd sit out on a third story patio
with a latte or cafe au lait and sip + stare.
I'd run or do something physical to feel better
about myself physically — maybe swim in a
nice big warm pool.
  Then I'd go visit something inspiring like a
museum or something. See great paintings. Something
to inspire. Then I'd hang glide peacefully down

December 4, 1999

1-28-00
Once again I sit at the fertility clinic with Allyson.

1-30-00
I'm not sure what to do about my hair. We
scanned in a picture of me + a dude with short

January 28, 2000

3-14-00
A heartbeat. I saw the baby's heartbeat. It was
pretty amazing. I will be a daddy. Hey dad, I'm gonna
join you + become a dad. I'm always late in the

March 14, 2000

63

4-3-00

So I sit once again in the Emory Clinic, waiting to be poked and prodded. CT scan, chest x-ray, bloodwork. Standard fare for the follow up cancer patient. Weird wild wacky stuff.

Yuck yuck yuck. This drink stuff is definitely the worst it has tasted. Gross gross. I wish the yuck in the back of my throat would go away.

April 3, 2000

4-9-00

Wow how things can change in a few days. Now I am on a plane to NYC and we've missed our chance at getting to Greece today. We've split up from Jill + Richard, as we've found out, for no reason since there were two seats left on this flight. BUT worst of all, I have a growth in my lung. Not what I was expecting at all. Now we're talking another operation. And chemotherapy. I hope we make it to Greece tomorrow. Please please please. I need it SO MUCH! And I don't want to blow a jillion dollars

April 4, 2000

4-30-00

It hath been two weeks since I have written in here. Since I last wrote I went to Istanbul, and I've had a major operation. I am in pretty serious pain right now, even though I've just taken narcotics. This kinda sux. I'm feeling low + grumpy.

April 30, 2000

5-8-00

What a shock; here I sit in a doctor's waiting room. And now I'm not. I am sitting back on my front porch. My staples are out. I feel fat. I can't wait to get back into shape. I'm a little nervous about chemo. I need to call Jonathan back. I missing doing it. I

May 8, 2000

5-28-00

There has got to be a good way to deal with chemo. Better than how I am dealing with it. Foods do not taste too good. I wonder if eggs would be good? I had such yucky dreams last night. The worst was waking up, after I had been out at this bizarro place that was a cross between a place in Ia and an abandoned restroomy kinda place. when I got home, I slept in my bed in PA. I woke up all wrapped up in a large bullwinkle. It was 4PM, sun was shining. It was pretty. I couldn't put on my glasses - it was as it the glasses or my face were completely out of whack. Finally, I'm in the bathroom, looking at myself in the mirror, my glasses a strange hodgepodge of these big brown ones with some string like Ali's necklace coming from it. So I decide to shake my head hard to shop out of it and I do exactly that. Back into reality. I realize my head was half squished on my pillow + that was why I couldn't get my glasses on, but much much worse, I was back, back in the the hell of chemo. I was so disheartened - it was such an incredible

May 28, 2000

7-9-00

Ali will probably be home soon. I had a great talk with Ali's mom that was very cool. All about letting go, living in the moment, expressing what is real, being creative, viewing work as art, it was uplifting. I really really want to finish the songs in the musical. The chemo song can be about all the side effects, the medicines for the side effects of the medicines for the side effects of medicines. There's only one way to get rid of him and that's poison. We must poison him, we must but to do so we must poison you. You must be strong and be able to fight it better than him. Ali's song. What about me? Why did this have to happen to him, to us? I don't care about some baby, I care about him. I don't want to be alone. Sometimes I feel like It'll be we'll be fine - this is just a minor detour. We're lucky. We'll get through it and we'll be ok. Sometimes it doesn't feel that way. What if he doesn't get better, what if he gets worse? What if we battle this for years and it slowly eats away at him, at us? It's such an unknown. And I want to know. I want to know + I want it to be good. This is not how my life is supposed to be. There are good ideas for the song. I must remember to go back and put these in. What about have a ball? What'll it take to make me better? What'll it take to make this end? What must we take to find out better what it'll take so that I'll mend? They say I only need one. They say they must take one to find out about it all more. Well if that is what it takes then I've got one thing to say, Have a Ball. Oh yes this is a great start. My god this is what I need. this is what I'm about This is the stuff I crave. It's what makes me alive. I live to create this stuff. I love to write the songs in this musical. I love to talk about living in the

July 9, 2000 - page 1

moment. (How can I teach others how to do it? Of course, I don't know entirely myself. But I'm getting better. Let go. Let it happen. Point + walk in the right direction. Even if it's hard and there are obstacles in the way. Climb over them do what it takes because it's all we get. Go toward the dream. ~~what~~ Watch for doors that open and WALK THRU THEM. Don't shoot for the 100% solution and spend all your energy getting there without moving at all. Figure out how you can get 5% or 10% better and get there. Now take what you've learned and go the next 5% or 10%. Eventually you will get to 95% and you will get there faster and better than if you shot for 100% out of the gate. You will also realize where the appropriate cutoff is. 95% tends to be pretty great and the effort to get to 100% from there is disproportionate and typically not worth it.

There. I've written some of the wisdom I've gained. The musical has been an idea. A thought about the direction. The big picture. A thought about the 100% but with no idea what it takes to get there and how best to go about it. Then I pointed myself and started walking in the right direction. I climbed over the obstacle of the first song. I went forward one song or idea at a time. I wrote what I knew and kept walking. I'd get 5-10% then move toward the next slowly gaining an better understanding of where 100% was. 1/16 = 1/16 x .625% per song. I'd let go and let the stuff happen. This musical is a manifestation of the wisdom I've gained up until this point in my life. That makes me feel like it will only get better. I am excited about life and how best to live it. Let go. Have direction. Walk toward it. Watch for ~~doors~~ opening. AES + Turning Thirty.

Back in the infusion center again. Nausea slowly creeping in, literally & figuratively. Must keep a good attitude. Can't forget about the musical ideas from a few days ago. I hope that I will feel better this time around. I hope I can keep a good outlook this week. I'm already feeling the nausea. Nausea. oops. spelling it wrong. I think. I hope I can eat ok. I hope I can feel good.

July 11, 2000

I'm sitting for day 2 of 5 in the infusion center, hell week. No major nausea yet. I'll be happy when it's over. I can't get over how much medicine gets pumped into me. I'm already feeling a little not so hot. Zip. It's next wednesday and I am being till nausea. We are beginning to stop the feeling of helplessness and ill-will. I can concentrate on baby again. Get the room up to shape. Dressers, paint, mouldings, crib, daybed, rocking chair, tables, rug, curtains. Lots money yet to spend. Poor lady next to me is not doing so well

August 1, 2000

8-7-00

I don't feel great, but I had my reawakening this morning. Somewhere between 5-7 AM right around sunrise, I cried. For the first time in since March, I actually felt as though the end were near. I imagine signs on the freeway where I've been on a detour through construction for hundreds of miles that say "Construction ends 45 miles" or "End of detour 50 miles". I picture the scene in "Groundhog Day" where Bill Murray says "It happened." Right now, instead of being overwhelmed by all this imagery, I am overwhelmed by the little pink pills - Benadryl. I just gave myself the shot and it was fine, but the Benadryl sure is making me loopy. I can't even write very fast or well for that matter.

Funny I've developed a taste for cinnamon gum, which I always shied away from since it burns my mouth. Now I feel more like "burn away" I feel alive. It is so temporary in comparison to other things I've felt that I actually enjoy the warm attempt at intensity.

I'm on the front porch, loopy, looking over at my work bench. Great stuff. I can't wait to set up my little shop down stairs. I should get a small extension cord and a heavy duty 6 outlet strip. I'll be able to finish up some projects pretty easily now.

Wow, the light at the end of the massive tunnel. It was in March when I got the news. It's now August, and I can finally see it. The dot showed up this morning - No

August 7, 2000 - page 1

big fanfare, no noise, no lights, not much of anything to do
except for the realization that yes indeed, for the first time,
there actually exists a light, a tiny hole at the end
of this hell tube which can no longer prevent light from
passing. I have seen the end, I now know it is not
solid but can and has been penetrated, a hole through which
nothing can prevent that glorious light from finding it's way
Quietly. It once was not there and suddenly it is. When
that realization arrived, neither could I stop the trickle of tears.
The tunnel I'm still in has taken a journey of four months to
get to the point where I no longer dream of the day when
it's no longer. I have seen it, I've felt it, I embraced it
I absorbed it. No army could prevent me from bursting out
to the other side.

I will make a production of crossing out "cure cancer"
on our chalkboard. I will celebrate that with friends,
family, and I will capture the event on film. I may never
know if it is actually gone, but I know that it will not
end me, I can beat it, I will beat it, and I will never
stop fighting it any + every time he comes around.
I now intend to help others even moreso than I have in the
past. I will make my job my mission. I will work hard
to ensure a healthy perspective so I can always keep good focus
+ direction to battling cancer and helping others prevent, cope, +
cure.

I will always strive to maintain good health. I will
take great care of the life I have, and I will do so for
the lives around me as well. I meditate and focus on life,
people, energy, integrity, perspective, wisdom. Whenever I feel
lost, overwhelmed, may the life + energy that binds all help
me to return to this place, where I can think clearly and
always walk in the right direction. I pray that if
I can come away from this experience with something truly
valuable, that it be this; the ability step back and

August 7, 2000 - page 2

always see the big picture. From there I can always
walk forward with confidence.

August 7, 2000 - page 3

saying that, but the real thing is to open the creativity
and let it flow. Have a Ball + Poison is left.

9-18-00

Here I sit in the waiting room at Dr. Staley's
office, no scratch that, actually I'm alone in an
exam room. I was just told that they will use a
local anesthesia, re-open the original incision, break up
the scar tissue and pull it out. A little spooky

September 18, 2000

So back to the musical.

Wizard wizard wizard wizard. Magic-lets do
word association. Magic wand Wizard Magician
Magician wizardry. Slight of hand. Science magic
dichotomy. Juxtaposition. Pointy hat. Stars moon.
Planets. Forces. The force. Jedi. Lightsaber. Sith.
Mystery. Appear. Disappear. Unbelievable. Awe-struck.
Belief challenging. Candles smoke. Transform. Shapes
Size. Fly. Soar. Rise. Float. Speed. Senses. Enhanced.
Motion. This is what I need to do musically creatively
I just need to make the ideas flow. Don't have

October 1, 2000

LYRICS

TURNING THIRTY - THE MUSICAL

CAST		SONGS
Tom	HERO	EVERYTHING'S COOL - Tom
ALLYSON	LOVE	YOUR NUMBER'S UP - T.C.
T.C.	EVIL DUDE	HOW COULD THIS BE - Tom
DIANA	ANGEL	WE WILL FACE THIS FOE - Dr. I.
DR. I.	FORCES OF GOOD	GET THROUGH THIS WITH YOU - Tom + ALI
		NOT DONE YET - T.C.
		I'm HERE FOR YOU - ANGEL + Tom
		EVERYTHING'S COOL AGAIN - ALL

Scene 1 - surprise 30th birthday party - complete w/ play within a play

last scene - baby

one theme / subplot - having a baby

SONG - FOR A CHILD - one time _not_ ready for a child
later   I am ready - " "
or CODA

first For a child is like a ....

later For this child I'd ...

Not Done Yet - You may try to get through this mother
but I'm not through with you
(*chorus)

Original show idea

72

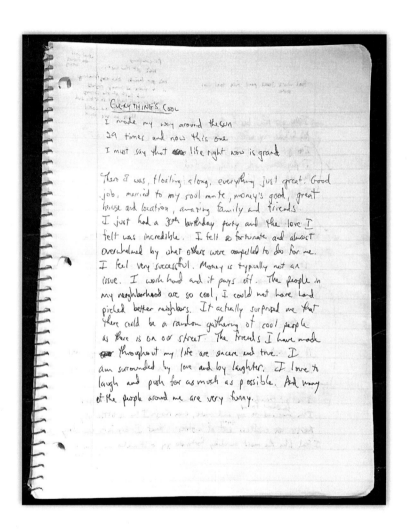

Life is Good, version 1 - Everything's Cool

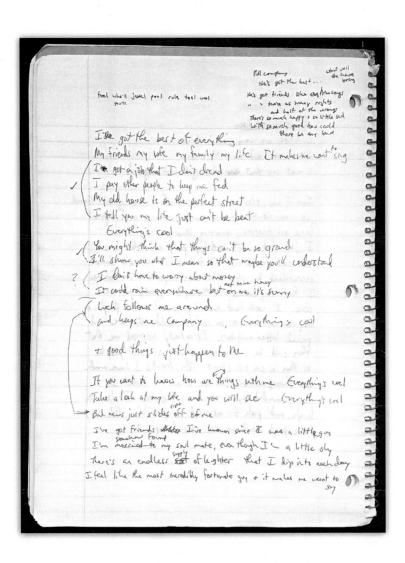

Life is Good, version 2 - Everything's Cool

Your Number's Up

Things have been going so well for so long. Almost too
well. I've been very healthy for 30 years and suddenly
bamm@! Here's some cancer. Cancer! For Christ's
sake, the very same shit that drained the life
from my father. Now it's in me

Things have gone so well for you   Too Well   Too Well
Time to cast a spell on you   Time to give you hell
But what could be the reason for this sudden turn for the worse
No reason is required if the cause is unknown   its just a curse
Because Your Number's Up   it's time for you to sweat
Yes   "   "   "   Yes thirty's all you get
That's more than you deserved   I hate to wait so long
Why should everything be so right when there is wrong

Look at you   Feeling everything is grand
A little bit of blue   can be placed neatly in your head
shit can hit you right there where you stand
When you least suspect it   you won't see it on its way   what it will be
But you'll know it ever it's there and you'll be too afraid to see   say
that
You have so much that's right so here's some wrong

Your Number's Up

75

How Could This Be

Everything was fine, everything was good
Now there's only rubble where great buildings once stood
My life has changed
I've lost my footing, my bearings
The pages of this my life neatly written
(now) are tearing
How Could This Be
I had no reason to believe that this would happen to me
The world I once knew is no longer true
And the one that I'm left with is so frightening to see
How Could This Be
Others have their problems, I once had those too
Now I'd gladly trade mine for theirs if that's what I could be
I used to be so healthy, I used to have it made
Now I feel as though I have some mysterious debt to be repaid

How dare this be the case What gall to mess with me
I've never hurt another at least not intentionally
He's come into my life and turned it upside down
What nerve of him to enter my peaceful little town

I am hurt I am bitter + for the life of me
I cannot see how this could be

How Could This Be

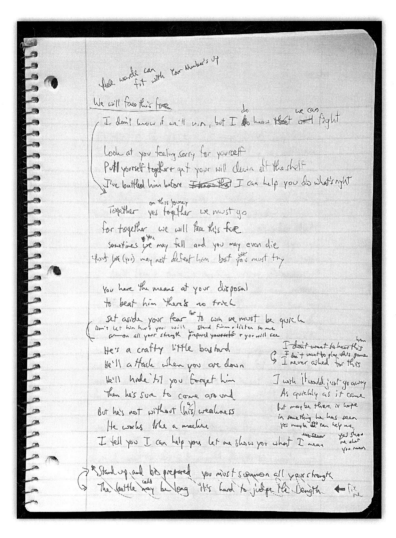

We Will Face This Foe

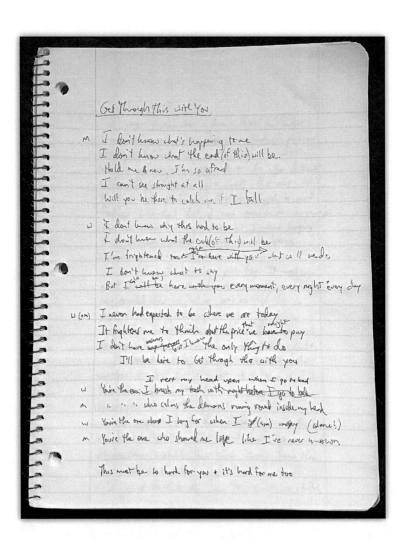

Get Through This With You

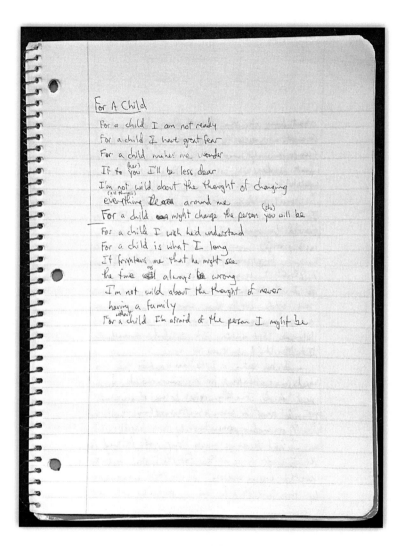

For a Child

who is this person   why is she so good to me

I'm Here For You

She knows exactly what to say, exactly what
to do. She's an angel I'm here for you She
gets me what I need, lets me do what I should do.
She takes care of things for me . I'm here for you
She appears when I need her. She's kind,
compassionate, generous. She keeps me sane,
She listens to me She helps me heal

I know you're hurting I can ease your pain
I know you're frightened I can help you save
Your battle's almost over Its time for you to rest
Though you may feel cursed Realize you're blessed

She appears when I need her she listens to me
                                              compels
She helps me to heal She helps me to see
That I am not beaten all is not lost
            must   has
I can move on despite what this cost
                  one way
I can forge ahead with so much behind me
I had felt lost now I can find me

I go when I am needed that's why I'm here with you
I can comfort you + help you heal because that is what I do
                                     you are
You may feel isolated but you're not alone
If you need strength I have some to give
Think of where you want to be then take that first step
You are not defeated you have the will the strength
     to bounce back you must stand you must walk you will live

I'm Here For You

The Best Job in the World

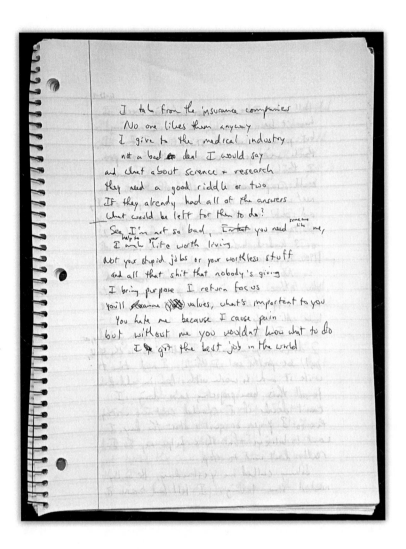

I take from the insurance companies
No one likes them anyway
I give to the medical industry
not a bad deal I would say
and what about science + research
they need a good riddle or two
If they already had all of the answers
What would be left for them to do?
See I'm not so bad, I that you need someone like me,
        help to your
I make life worth living
Not your stupid jobs or your worthless stuff
and all that shit that nobody's giving
I bring purpose I return focus
you'll reexamine values, what's important to you
You hate me because I cause pain
but without me you wouldn't know what to do
        I got the best job in the world

The Best Job in the World - page 2

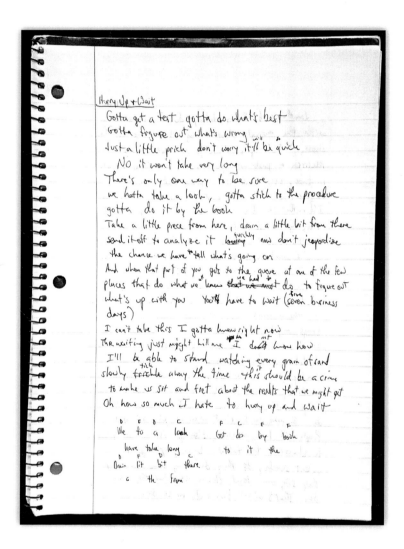

Hurry Up and Wait

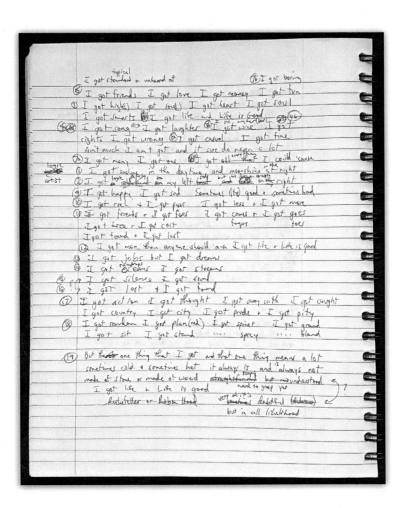

Life is Good Finale

Life is Good

I got sunshine in the daytime and moonshine in the night
I got logic on my left side but an artist on my right
I got high I got low I got heart I got soul
I got friends? I got love I got typical & unheard of
I got everything I could I got life & Life is Good
I got higher & I got lower I got right & I got wrong
I got many I got one I got boring I got fun
I got casual I got fine I got water I got wine
I got happy I got sad sometimes good & sometimes bad
I got rich & I got poor I got less & I got more
I got friends & I got foes I got comes & I got goes
I got more than anyone should 'cause I got life & Life is Good

I got jobs but I got dreams I got raindrops I got streams
I got silence I got sound I got lost & I got found
I got action I got thought I got away with I got caught
I got random I got planned I got spin & I got grand

But there's one thing that I got and that one thing means a lot
Sometimes cold & sometimes hot It always is and is always not
hard to grasp yet understood very doubtful but in all likelihood
I got life and Life is Good

Life is Good Finale - page 2

There have been times in my life _I had no_
when I had myself no girlfriend let alone a wife
And there would be times
when I could cut the tension with a knife
I felt as though I had no control
I felt as though I'd sell my _(own)_ (very) soul
Just to snuff out the burning flame, to make the wild horses tame
To force the voices in my head to shut up, but I never thought I'd masturbate
in a cup

Masturbating in a cup feels very strange
will make a man change
Oh I've done this before, but one thing's for sure
I never had to stress about my aim
With a cup it's a completely new game _I may never be the same (feel)_
I had to watch where it went when I come

I consider myself a sensitive man
but they got magazines and videos to help out my hand
Other men I know are so jealous of me
I get to leave work _early_ and watch pornography
Not only that but I can do so with impunity _to look at_
So why do I feel like everyone's looking at me
staring

(when)
Well the room is so bland and yet sterile
It doesn't really make make me feel virile
I do this _here_ so that later we can always have kids _to make sure that_
I just hope they never ask about what daddy did

C C C C | C F C C F G C C C F C C F G C C⁷
F G E^m A^m D^m G C C⁷ F G E⁷ A^m D⁷ D⁷ G E⁷ F G C
(Chorus→) C⁷ F G C C⁷ F G A^m A^m F C E⁷ A^m D⁷ D⁷ G G⁷ F G C (C)
C F G C F G C C⁷
F G E^m A^m D^m G C C⁷ F G E⁷ A^m D⁷ D⁷ G G⁷
repeat Chorus
F G C C F G C C F G E⁷ A^m D⁷ D⁷ G G⁷
repeat Chorus

Masturbating in a Cup

Fight Song

We meet again

Yes it's true. Why do you keep doing what you do

Why do I ... You must grow tired of facing me
No matter what you seem to do I've come back for him
or perhaps you

I don't care what you say You won't win not today

He was never an easy mark, I can keep you in the dark

I must warn you his will is strong Together we'll make sure
you're gone.

I grow tired of this senseless chatter let's get to
the heart of the matter
Try to stop me or get out of my way

Oh we will stop you (and) you will pay

I will pay don't brake me laugh insult me
I've made you both pay already don't you see

/ You know it's true but are so afraid to see

We're strong are prepared you will see

   because your number's up it's time for you to sweat
      Together the journey's led us here
   yes your number's up and thirty's all you get
      Together the end is very near
   But's more than you deserved I hate to wait so long
      we must strike before long
   why should everything be so right
      if he thinks he'll win
   why should everything be so tight
      if he thinks he'll win
   when there is wrong
      he is wrong

The Battle

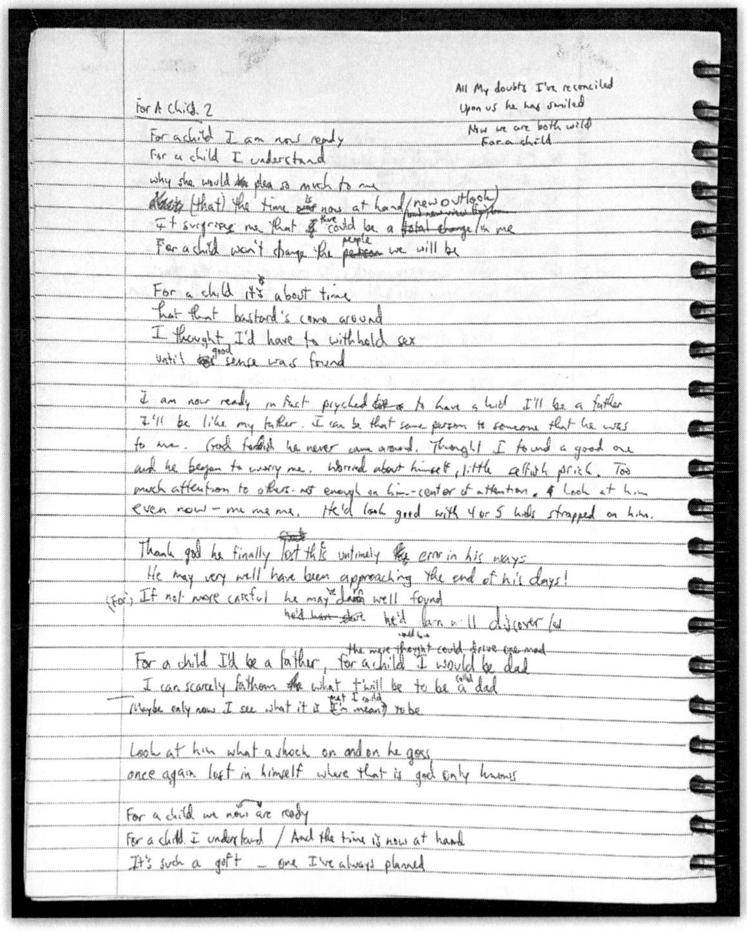

Handwritten notebook page:

All My doubts I've reconciled
Upon us he has smiled

Now we are both wild
For a child

For A Child 2

For a child I am now ready
For a child I understand

why she would plea so much to me
~~Knowing~~ (that) the time is now at hand / (new outlook)
It surprise me that I ~~five~~ could be a ~~total change~~ / in me
For a child won't change the ~~pattern~~ people we will be

For a child it's about time
that that bastard's come around
I thought I'd have to withhold sex
until good sense was found

I am now ready in fact psyched ~~for~~ to have a child. I'll be a father
I'll be like my father. I can be that same person to someone that he was
to me. God ~~forbid~~ he never came around. Thought I found a good one
and he began to worry me. Worried about himself, little selfish prick. Too
much attention to others, not enough on him. center of attention, & look at him
even now — me me me. He'd look good with 4 or 5 kids strapped on him.

Thank god he finally lost this untimely ~~flag~~ error in his ways.
He may very well have been approaching the end of his days!
(For:) If not more careful he may well in well found
he'd burn all discover /u

For a child I'd be a father, the more thought could drive one mad
for a child I would be dad
I can scarcely fathom ~~the~~ what t'will be to be a dad
Maybe only now I see what it is ~~that I told~~ I'm meant to be

Look at him what a shock on and on he goes
once again lost in himself where that is god only knows

For a child we now are ready
For a child I understand / And the time is now at hand
It's such a gift — one I've always planed

For a Child 2

Have a Ball - page 1

Ali's song

Sometimes I stand, sometimes I fall. Sometimes I wonder
if anyone understands at all. ← a capella
// What about me? Why did this have to happen to him, to us? I don't
care about some baby I care about him. I don't want to be
alone. // Sometimes I feel like we'll be fine - this is just a
minor detour. We're lucky, we'll get through it, and we'll be ok.
Sometimes it doesn't feel that way. / What if he doesn't get
better, what if he gets worse? What if we battle this for years
and it slowly eats away at him, at us? It's such an unknown,
and I want to know. I want it to be known and I want it
to be good. This is not how my life is supposed to be. // I'd
have a husband who loves me and treats me well. We'd have carloads
of children with stories to tell. Learning and growing and caring
yearning and going and sharing. This is the way it was meant to
be, not the way it turned out for me // ① I can't stand to see
him this way. ② I don't want to live if he's not here, too
③ Tired and pained + suffering all day. ④ I think of what might be
and don't know what to do. // (This is killing me too.)
What's worse is the man I can turn to, & can lean on
when I keep in pain, is the one who can't help me, the one
who's in pain. Dear god what on earth am I supposed
to do? ←

Sometimes - page 1

Poison

Poison. Side effects. Anal fissure. Loss of senses. hearing, energy,
smelling, tasting, touching. Rash. Tender fingers. Sores
in mouth. Painful swallows. Nausea. Tired. Depression.
Sight sound(hearing) Taste touch smell. All your senses go to hell
Bruises. Hair loss. Bald. steroid pear shape. No immune
system. Bone pain. Wash your hands. Emotional ball of mush.
Watch for fevers. Medicines for the side effects of medicines for
the side effects of medicines. There's only one way to get
rid of him and that's poison. We must poison him, and
to do that we must poison you. You must be strong
and be able to fight it better than him.
I ain't talk I can't smell and my hearing's gone to hell   six months
Cut me up cut it out you'll heal you'll be fine in six weeks at the most
But just to be sure we must poison the host to kill the parasite
Hurts to swallow I can't eat painful fingers and bruised feet
I feel sick, must lie down don't dehydrate while you drown
Hurts to piss hurts to shit Too sick to stand too sore to sit
Don't get a fever can't fight it now can't stop never don't know how   coughing
pills for the side effects of pills for the side effects of pills
bills for the poisons and pills but no pills for the bills
Give yourself shots get pain in your bones
no one knows your goals no one hears your moans
because the only way to be sure is with poison
well, mostly sure
Lose my hair everywhere fight depression with despair
sleep all day + up all night a terrible rash that I can't fight
there's got to be a better way maybe they'll come up with one some day
but until then I have no choice
even if I shout with my scratchy voice
well the only way to be mostly sure
"   "   "   somewhat sure is with poison

lose your appetite then put on weight try to stick to the schedule but you're
                                                                gonna be late

Poison - page 1

91

Poison

all share with you   to make this one a ghost
① I know the answer. I don't wish to boast
here it is: to kill the parasite we must poison the host   all you need to do is
sleep all day up all night
there's got to be a better way, maybe they'll come up with one someday
but until then I have no choice
even if I shout with my scratchy voice
controlled poisoning - kill off part of me

He wants to feeds off of you he can't exist without you   wizard
① I've analyzed him I know what he needs
He can't exist without you, it's off you he feeds
So if you want him off your back you've come to the right place
I can make him go away, disappear without a trace

I know the secret formula I have the magic potion
"settle down relax, no cause for a commotion

I can't see, I can't hear My hearing's gone to hell
Too sick to stand too sore to sit to all this torture I submit
pain in my skin pain in my bones, no one knows my aches, no one hears my moans
I sleep all day up all night just too much for me to fight

I pray this works I hope he's right (prays)
'cause At the end of this clearly tunnel I have yet to see a (the) light
The only way to be sure, well the only way to be mostly sure
is with poison

Don't you worry my troubled friend   soon all of this will end

is this for real
Nothing could assuage how horrible I feel

Poison - page 2

92

Sometimes / Killing me too

Sometimes I stand   Sometimes I fall
Sometimes I wonder if anyone understands at all

What about me
Why did this even have to happen at all
I don't care about some baby, I care about him
I don't want to be alone should he fall

Sometimes I feel like we will be fine
We're lucky, we'll get through it, and we'll be ok
This is just a minor detour
But sometimes it doesn't feel that way

What if it doesn't get better, what if it gets worse
What if we battle this for years until it finally breaks him and breaks me
    It's such an unknown and I want to know
    I want it to be known and I want it to be good
This is not how my life is supposed to be

I'd have a husband who loves me and treats me so well
We'd have carloads of children with stories to tell
    Learning and growing and caring
    Yearning and going and sharing
This is the way it was meant for me, not the way it turned out to be

I can't stand to see him this way
Tired and pained and suffering all day
I think of what might be and don't know what to do
I don't want to live if he's not here too

The worst part is the man I can turn to, can lean on, who keeps me sane
is the one who can't help me, the one who's in pain
Dear God what on earth am I supposed to do
This horrible nightmare is killing me too

Sometimes - page 2

93

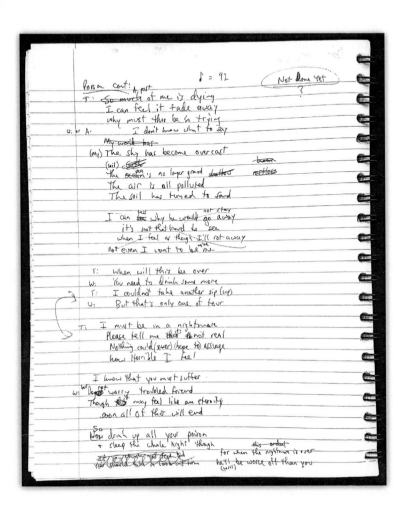

♩ = 92   Not Done Yet
?

Poison cont: A part

T: So much of me is dying
I can feel it fade away
why must this be so trying
u: or A: I don't know what to say

(my) The sky has become overcast
(will)
The ocean's no longer grand   restless
The air is all polluted
The soil has turned to sand

I can tell why he would go away   not stay
it's not that hard to see
when I feel as though I'll rot away
not even I want to be me

T: When will this be over
W: You need to drink some more
T: I couldn't take another sip (cup)
W: But that's only one of four

T: I must be in a nightmare
Please tell me this is not real
Nothing could (ever) (hope to) assuage
how horrible I feel!

I know that you must suffer.
W: Don't worry troubled friend
Though this may feel like an eternity
soon all of this will end

So
Now drink up all your poison
+ sleep the whole night though   for when the nightmare is over
he'll be worse off than you
(will)

Poison - page 3

94

Have a Ball
I used to think they'd always be around
No reason to think otherwise I'd found
Then one day everything had changed
And my thoughts on the subject were completely rearranged

It occurred to me that something had gone wrong
And I'd have to act to fix it before long
I had little time I had to make the call
So I thought why should I worry when I can just have a ball

Have a Ball Have a Ball Oh I'm up against a wall
If I let them have a ball there's only one left yes that's all
They say I need just one, they say it won't hurt at all
Well if that's what it takes then baby have a ball

Now you might think that it's an easy choice
And you would not be afraid to raise your voice
But let me tell you it's not simple at all, no
When you're face to face with the decision to have a ball

Oh it's scary yes its very solitary makes me wary
like an unnecessary adversary it seems so involuntary
why am I the only guy who's happy life's gone so awry
I used to be tough, I used to stand tall
I used to have balls but now I only have a ball

Though well if that's what it takes
though it gives me the shakes
please don't make any mistakes and baby
Have a Ball

Have a Ball - page 2

95

Not Done Yet

① We (they) think that I'm defeated
   * they think (that) I'm ~~am~~ gone (for good)
② they think they killed me with a blade   the blade had slain me
   I'm ~~not~~ sure they ~~think~~ they could   ② I'm so misunderstood
        ~~though it~~ should

But I am Not Done Yet
~~Remember~~ Don't underestimate me
        Yet I'll be back
        Just you wait and see
No I'm Not Done Yet   I'm just laying out of sight
   → No not quite thought   but
   Rather   If you think that this is over was
   for. I've just begun to fight   you will wish that you were right
        * Don't go thinking this is over

Don't go thinking it am thru
        without a fight

Not Done Yet

96

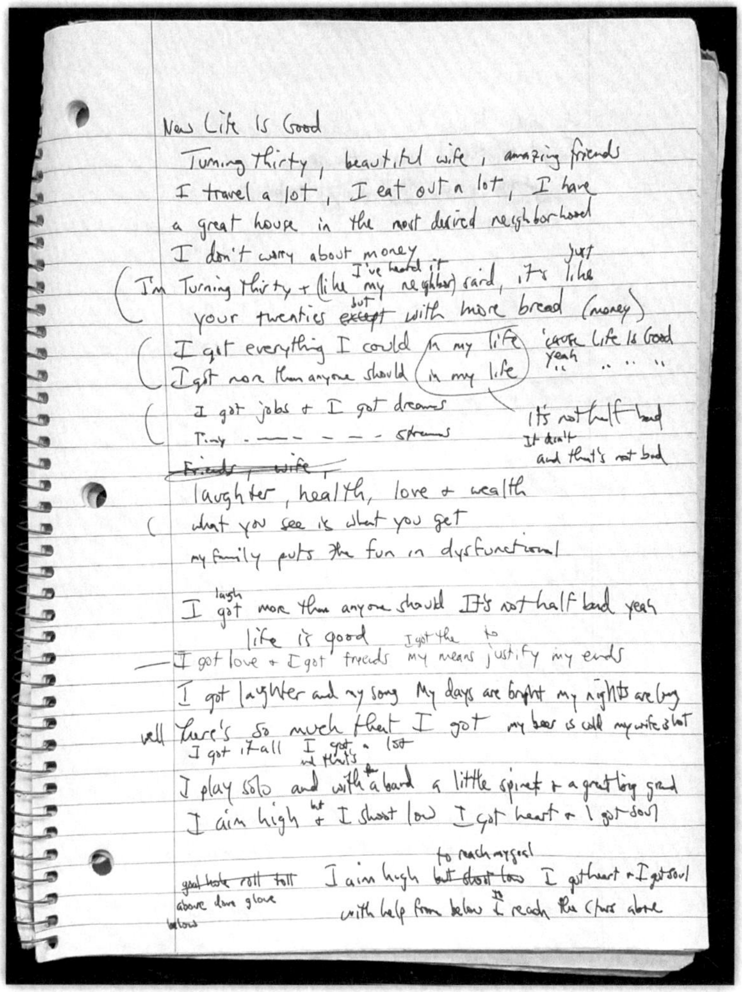
New Life Is Good
Turning Thirty, beautiful wife, amazing friends
I travel a lot, I eat out a lot, I have
a great house in the most desired neighborhood
I don't worry about money
I'm Turning Thirty & like I've heard it my neighbor said, it's just like
your twenties ~~except~~ but with more bread (money)
I got everything I could in my life 'cause Life Is Good yeah
I got more than anyone should in my life " " " "
I got jobs & I got dreams
Tiny - - - - - - streams
It's not half bad
It don't
and that's not bad
~~Friends, wife,~~
laughter, health, love & wealth
what you see is what you get
my family puts the fun in dysfunctional
I laugh got more than anyone should It's not half bad yeah
life is good
I got love & I got friends I got the to my means justify my ends
I got laughter and my song My days are bright my nights are long
well there's so much that I got my beer is cold my wife is hot
I got it all I got a lot and that's
I play solo and with the a band a little spinet & a great big grand
I aim high but & I shoot low I got heart & I got soul
~~goal hole~~ roll toll I aim high ~~but shoot low~~ to reach my goal I got heart & I got soul
above dove glove below with help from below to I reach the stars above

Life is Good - new opening version

MEDICAL

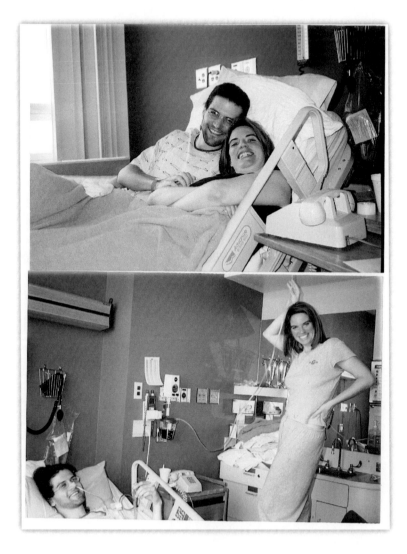

*Retroperitoneal lymph node dissection
(RPLND) operation*

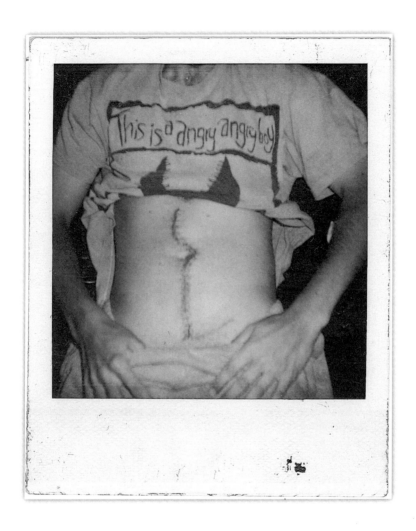

RPLND Scar

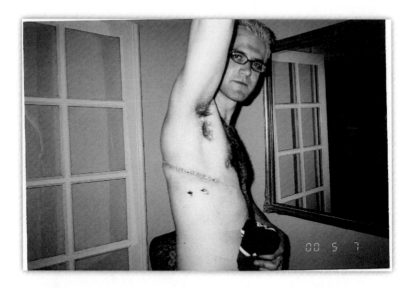

Lung Thoracotomy

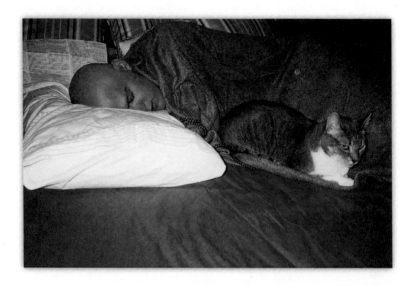

Chemo

PRESS

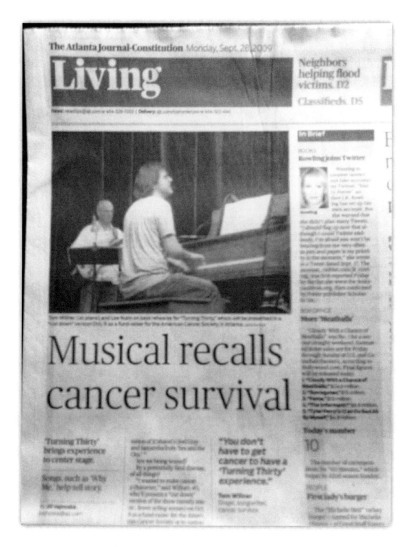

Atlanta Journal-Constitution (AJC) article

Cancer survivor writes musical about disease

'Turning Thirty' is a portrayal of what cancer survivor experiences.

By Ann Hardie
For the AJC

A diagnosis of cancer doesn't generally cause people to break into song. But that's what Tom Willner did after learning he had testicular cancer on the cusp of his thirtieth birthday. In fact, he wrote a whole musical about it. "I've always been a musician. One of the ways that I dealt with the whole ordeal was to write it to music," said Willner, whose day job coincidentally is director of web development for the American Cancer Society. Over the past five years, "Turning Thirty, The Musical" has played in various venues at various times for various charitable causes around town. Now 43 and cancer free for some time, Willner has raised $10,000 and is making a big push to get the musical picked up by a local or regional theater. This coming week, the Virginia Highland resident is hosting a workshop with theater professionals, followed by a June 10 showcase performance that is free and open to the public. For more on Willner's journey with cancer, and the musical it inspired, visit turningthirty.org.

Q: Who wants to see a musical about cancer?
A: Cancer affects nearly everyone in some way, and the subject has become less and less taboo. People have become more willing to address it for what it is – a health problem that we need to get rid of. Plus, the musical not only addresses cancer but getting older. My wife and I didn't have kids at the time so cancer brought that discussion to the forefront.

Q: You conceived three children through in vitro fertilization. Were you worried that you weren't going to be around for them?
A: There is a scene in the musical that touches on this. My wife said she always wanted to have kids and she wanted to have kids with me. If I lost my battle with cancer, she said, there would be a piece of me in them. That really struck a chord with me.

Q: Did cancer fundamentally change your

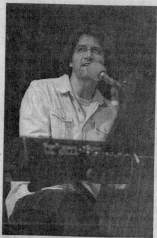

Tom Willner, cancer survivor, musician and web director at the American Cancer Society, performs during his musical, "Turning Thirty."
CONTRIBUTED BY TOM WILNER

IF YOU GO
What: "Turning Thirty, The Musical"
When: 7:30 to 9:30 p.m., June 10
Where: Theatrical Outfit Balzer Theater, 84 Luckie St. N.W., Atlanta
Cost: Free
Information: turningthirty.eventbrite.com

does lend itself to jokes. Humor played a big part for me dealing with cancer.

Q: You work for the American Cancer Society. You are pushing your musical about cancer. Don't you worry about tempting fate?
A: My wife and I have always had a "to do" list. There's the standard stuff on there like yard work. After cancer, we added things like

AJC second article

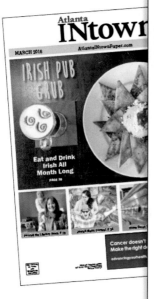

PLAYWRIGHT, SOCIAL WORKER BRING CANCER MUSICAL TO NATIONAL AUDIENCE

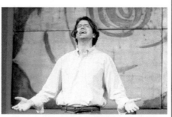

Tom Willner, above and bottom photo, wrote "Turning Thirty" after his own bout with cancer. Anne McSweeney, middle, is helping to bring it to a national audience.

By Clare S. Richie

Atlanta playwright and cancer survivor Tom Willner will perform "Turning Thirty," an acclaimed musical about his cancer experience, at the prestigious World Congress of Continuing Professional Development in San Diego later this month.

"I've always wanted my show to help others understand cancer from the patient's perspective," said Willner.

Last June, Anne McSweeney, a social worker and founder of CEU Concepts (an acronym for Creative, Educational, Unique) called Willner with just such an opportunity.

Healthcare professionals such as doctors, nurses and social workers must obtain a certain number of continuing education hours on a yearly basis in order to keep up their license. Many earn their credit hours from standard lectures and presentations. With a musical and interactive discussion afterward – an extremely unique stage is set for the participant to learn.

McSweeney spent over 15 years working closely with geriatric clients throughout the Atlanta area. She was required to take continuing education classes, which were expensive and often boring. In 2010, she founded CEU Concepts in a light bulb moment. She would bring in sponsors to drive down or eliminate attendance fees and would develop creative and interactive workshops.

Ever since McSweeney read about Willner's "Turning Thirty" several years ago, she'd thought about by pairing it

with a healthcare team discussion. So, last June, when a speaker cancelled due to illness for an event with 90 registrants, McSweeney decided it was time to put her idea to the test.

Willner jumped at the opportunity. He performed a solo version of his musical, staying in character and talking to the audience between songs. During the discussion that followed, attendees remained engaged.

"Tom stepped right in and our collaboration and synergy was instant – a perfect format for learning," said McSweeney. "This was a continuing education course that attendees will remember, especially with a take home musical CD."

From there, McSweeney submitted the proposal that was accepted at the World Congress of Continuing Professional Development, which she says opens the door to more possibilities.

"We want to take the show on the road. Get into hospitals around the US. or "franchise" the program so that others could perform it across the country," shared Willner and McSweeney.

Willner also submitted "Turning Thirty" to theaters across the US. and is expecting to hear back shortly. Regardless of the avenue, he expects his future to include pursuit of his dual passions of music and addressing cancer.

"My hope is that with this unique event we've created, we'll be able to provide healthcare professionals with a deeper understanding of the cancer experience, and ultimately benefit cancer patients and their families across the country," said Willner.

AtlantaINtownPaper.com

Atlanta Intown article

SHOWS

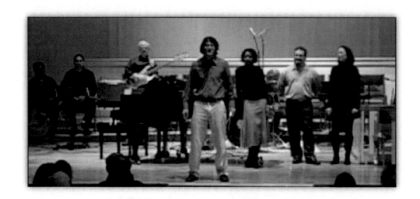

2008 Debut Performance

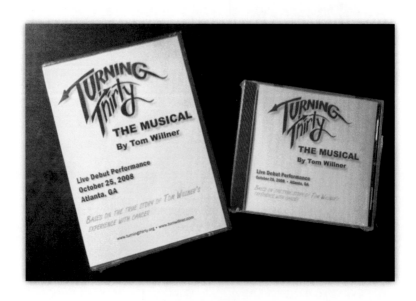

CD and DVD

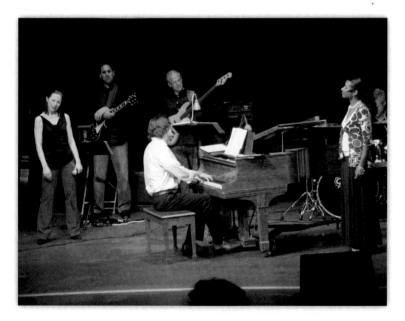

2009 Second Performance

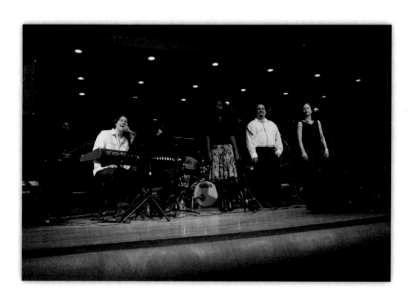

2009 Third Performance

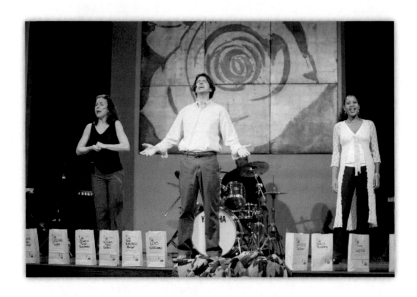

2010 Fourth Performance

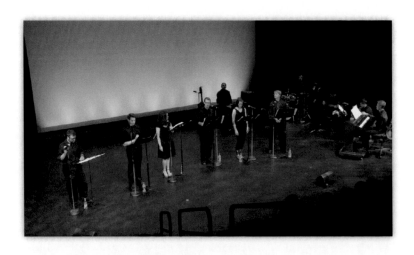

2013 Workshop Showcase

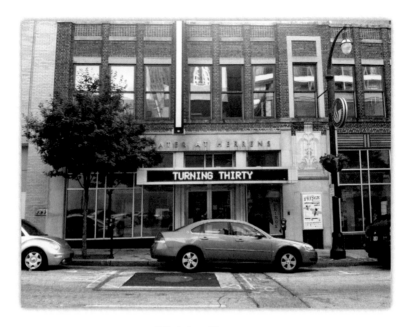

Workshop Showcase

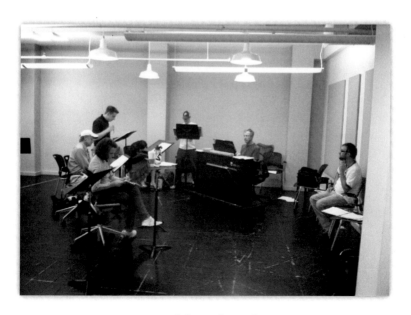

Workshop Rehearsal

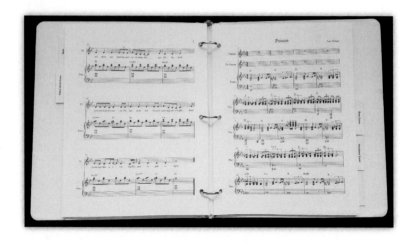

Sheet music developed for the workshop

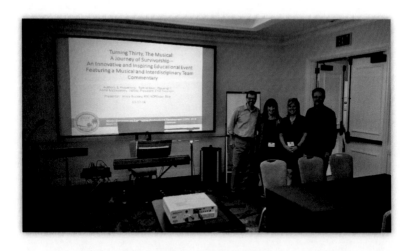

2016 Presentation at the
World Congress on Continuing
Professional Development

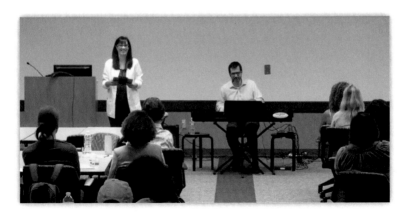

2016 Center Stage Education event

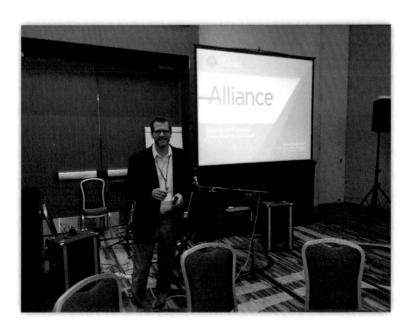

2017 Presentation at the Alliance for
Continuing Education in the Health Professions

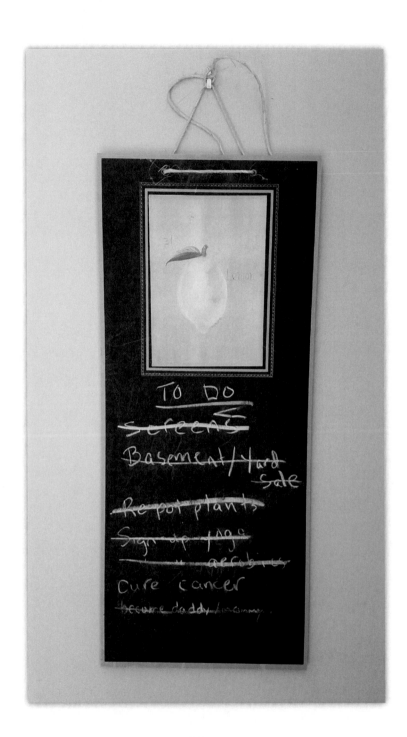

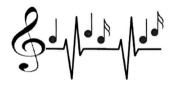

LIFE IS GOOD (TWO VERSIONS)

*"I realize that every single living, breathing moment
is one to be savored, no matter whether it is easy or difficult,
good or bad, right or wrong."*

~ Tom Willner

"Comedy and Tragedy are roommates..."

~ Gilbert Gottfried

*"All the world's a stage, And all the men and women merely
players; They have their exits and their entrances, And one
man in his time plays many parts..."*

~ William Shakespeare, from Act 2 of *'As You Like It'*

I COME BACK TO the song that started it all for me. Here I need to do a sort of flashback.

Right from the time I wrote the words "Turning Thirty" at the top of that page in my journal — the two words that spawned this whole musical — I knew that I had to write the main song. I knew this was going to be the main song, the opening and closing paragraph to my thesis.

This was one of the most difficult songs to write. I wanted it to sum up the whole experience. I visited and revisited this song, over and over. I had to look at the whole experience from above, which looked a little like this.

INSPIRATION

At the time when my 30th birthday was coming around in 1999, when I discovered the lump on my testicle and booked the doctor exam, the first thing I wrote down in my notebook (as a musician taking notes and jotting ideas) was "Turning Thirty — The Musical." Then on the left side, I wrote "Cast" with 5 characters (including TC and other characters I kept), and on the right side I wrote "Songs" with 8 song titles and who would sing them. The entire idea for the musical was downloaded to me in one journal entry, in one inspired moment from above. All the songs became numbers for the musical with those exact titles, except this one. Originally, I envisioned two versions of this song which I called "Everything's Cool" and "Everything's Cool Again."

After that opening salvo, I tried to write "Everything's Cool." Unfortunately, I just couldn't figure out the right words to say, so I moved on to the next song. I kept in mind that the song in two versions would be a good open and close to a story like this. It is a, "Tell 'em what you're gonna say, say it, and then tell 'em what you told 'em" sort of song. The song would change for the closing version depending on how the Conlan character evolved throughout his healing journey.

THE OPEN AND THE CLOSE

I made at least 3 attempts at this song before I got to one I liked. After writing several streams of consciousness about how my life was then, things came together as a demonstration of my view that my life really was good. I finally completed the lyrics to my satisfaction and settled on the title "Life is Good."

In a somewhat ironic twist, it was on April 3, 2000, the day I got the fateful CT scan that found my recurrence of cancer, when I journaled "the new song rocks." I was referring to 'Life is Good'.

I actually crafted all the other songs before I was fully finished with both versions of this one. I think I needed to tell a whole story with song and script first to know how to introduce and conclude it. The first version of the song opens the story and the musical. A second version of it closes the show.

It turns out I wrote the finale version first, not the opening. The finale is the version where I already had my new perspective on life. At first, I used the same lyrics for the opening version, just with a different musical style.

In the "it was destined to be" vein of thinking, I think nailing the finale version of this song before the opening version was probably a clue that I was being led by divine powers to a good conclusion of this experience with cancer. It was like holding my destination in mind with a firm commitment to getting there, in spite of not really knowing what kind of roller coaster ride was in store along the way.

Much later, when I did a professional workshop of the show, we decided the opening version needed to be more representative of someone prior to having a life-changing ordeal. When I was pre-cancerous and still in pre-diagnosis, I needed to say, "Life is GOOD," with the emphasis on "good." That's when I rewrote some lyrics to reflect the Life is GOOD approach at the beginning of the show, to portray things in the pre-diagnosis period.

For a long time, the music for the opener was very upbeat, and the finale version was slow and somber. Later, I changed the finale to start somber but become more upbeat with a big finish. Tempo plays a big role in communicating this song, its two versions and meanings. While the opener needed to say Life is *good*, at the end of the ordeal, I needed to say that *Life is Good*, with the emphasis on "life."

My friends didn't flee when I was diagnosed, when I needed them most. My wife stood by me in the hardest of dialogs with doctors. She stood with me through her own emotional moments, not to mention my own. I could still smile, joke, and laugh, though I also shouted through my share of tears. I got lost in the tragedy of death and dying. I found myself in the midst of joyous new parenthood, new life, and living.

From my observations all throughout the entire cancer experience, all the doctor visits, tests, and procedures, I had the two versions — the announcement of my journey and my return from the journey — of my song. Conlan's song.

LIFE IS GOOD

I got sunshine in the daytime and moonshine in the night.

I got logic on my left side and an artist on my right.

I got rock, I got roll, I got heart, and I got soul.

I got laughter and my song. My days are bright. My nights are long.

I got love and I got friends. I got means to justify my ends.

I got everything I could. It ain't half bad. Yeah, life is good.

I got travel across the sea, so many places that I got to be.

I got casual and fine. I got water and a whole lot of wine.

I got happy. I got mad, sometimes crazy, but always glad.

For every will there is some way. Sometimes work, sometimes play.

I'm turning thirty and I've heard it said, it's just like your twenties with a lot more bread.

I got more than anyone should. It ain't half bad. Yeah, life is good.

I got jobs, but I got dreams. Tiny raindrops make up streams.

I got silence within sound. I get lost but then I'm found.

I got action along with thought. I get away with, but I get caught.

I play solo and with the band, a little spinet and a great big grand,

But there's one thing that I got and that one thing means a lot.

Sometimes cold and sometimes hot, it always is and is always not.

Hard to grasp yet understood, very doubtful but in all likelihood

I'm living the good life. Yeah, life is good.

Life Is Good Finale

I got sunshine in the daytime and moonshine in the night.

I got logic on my left side and an artist on my right.

I got high. I got low.   got heart and I got soul.

I got laughter and my song. I got right. I got wrong.

I got friends and I got love. I got typical and unheard of.

I got everything I could 'cause I got life and life is good.

I got many for every one, a whole lot of boring, but a mess of fun.

I got casual and fine. I got water and a whole lot of wine.

I got happy. I got sad. Sometimes good and sometimes bad.

For every rich there is some poor. Sometimes less, sometimes more.

I got friends. I got foes. Easy comes and easier goes.

I got more than anyone should 'cause I got life and life is good.

I got jobs, but I got dreams. Tiny raindrops make up streams.

I got silence within sound. I get lost but then I'm found.

I got action along with thought. I get away with but I get caught.

I got random though it's planned, a little spinet and a great big grand,

But there's one thing that I got and that one thing means a lot.

Sometimes cold and sometimes hot, it always is and is always not

Hard to grasp yet understood very doubtful but in all likelihood

I got life and life is good.

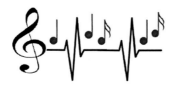

MASTURBATING IN A CUP

"In the early days, all I hoped was to make a living out of what I did best. But since there's no real market for masturbation, I had to fall back on my bass-playing abilities."

~ Les Claypool

"When my kids ask me where babies come from, I say, 'First, you call your embryologist.'"

~ Tom Willner

"If God had intended us not to masturbate, he would've made our arms shorter."

~ George Carlin

"Don't knock masturbation. It's sex with someone I love."

~ Woody Allen

I'D FINISHED UP YET another cheap drugstore notebook. I bought myself a nicer one to celebrate! Actually, it was spiral bound and college-ruled, very classy (I thought it was very punny at the time). I added more things to personalize it, according to *The Artist's Way*. I cut images that I liked from color magazines — stuff I found beautiful, interesting, or just happy — and pasted the covers and some of the pages with images of beauty. Mostly homes from *Architectural Digest* in beautiful locations — overlooking the ocean or suspended from a mountainside.

Coming from me, the practical, functional guy that I had been, this addition of beauty was new. I'd never had that kind of designed environment for myself. Maybe this was my version of nesting. I'd gotten a fortune in a fortune cookie that said, "You create your own stage; the audience is waiting," and I pasted it on the cover of my journal, too.

I had been recording the songs I had so far and burning CDs to share with a couple of close friends. Other songs came to me around this time, outside of this *Turning Thirty* theme. They usually never ended up being much of anything. I didn't do anything with most of them. On another musical note, I played the *Eddie's Attic* gig with my talented and good friend, Ben.

IDENTITY

Another notable thing going on around February was a sort of identity crisis. I had long, pony-tailed hair before my diagnosis and surgeries. The Grizzly Adams beard came after the surgery. At the first of the year, I got my hair cut for *Wigs for Kids*. It had been cut specifically over prior months so that I could make this donation. Then I bleached what was left blond. My wife said it was like sleeping with a new guy. It was quite a big event at work, too. The folks at work did double takes at the overnight change from dark ponytail to short blond. I walked by a meeting room window and a coworker waved — then bolted up to come and admire my new hair. Related, perhaps, to my nesting attempts, this was about trying to spark the creativity that I'd been tapping into since September.

The fact that Allyson had a miscarriage and had had time to recover, and that I was also much better recovered from surgery, got us thinking about pregnancy again. We'd done preparation for the in-vitro fertilization (IVF). It was around February 2000. Klara, our first child, was born in November, so obviously the IVF succeeded!

I think that moving back into baby-making mode helped me remember my prior summer experience of masturbating in a cup those two times at the clinic. As I wrote two more pages in my journal with various potential ideas for scenes and dialog for the musical, I had this masturbating in a cup experience in the back of my mind for a light-hearted song. The "in a cup" was the part I was going to poke fun at.

"Bopping the Baloney in a Cup" was a first song title. Obviously, that didn't make the cut. The title emerged as I wrote the words.

What was clear to me was that this just had to be a country song in a major key, with twangy guitars doing old-fashioned 3/4 country time, with some boompah-pah underlying beats involved. What's a funny twist is that the two female (rather than male) characters do back up and share a chorus with me, the lead singer. I've always liked the clever twist to the words that country songs tend to have. This was my attempt at a classic country twist. "I never had to stress about my aim." "I hope my kids never ask about what dear daddy did."

In August 1999, I had an appointment at the fertility clinic, and mentioned to a co-worker that I had to go to the fertility clinic (aka the sperm bank) and make a deposit. The look on his face and his reaction were priceless: "You get to leave work on company time to do that?!" Yup, I got to leave work early and watch pornography — the guys would be jealous of me. I'd made two deposits in the summer, before my surgery, but that was to be it for my sperm — forever more.

In the lyrics, I'm dancing around the fact of a sexual act, that building of sexual tension without someone as an outlet for it. Without my wife with me. Shame and a certain amount of embarrassment are a part of the whole experience, in a fun kind of way. Frankly, it doesn't make a guy feel virile in such a sterile environment. Conlan sings.

MASTURBATING IN A CUP

There have been times in my life
When I had myself no girlfriend and I had no wife
And there would be times
When I could cut the tension with a knife.
I felt as though I had no control.
I felt as though I'd sell my own soul
Just to snuff out the burning flame,
To make the wild horses tame,
To force the voices in my head to shut up,
But I never thought I'd masturbate in a cup.
Masturbating in a cup feels very strange.
Masturbating in a cup will make a man change.

Oh I've done this before, but one thing's for sure.
I never had to stress about my aim.
With a cup, it's a completely new game.
I consider myself a sensitive man.

But they got magazines and videos to help out my hand.
Other men I know are so jealous of me.
I get to leave work early and watch pornography.
Not only that, but I can do so with impunity,
So why do I feel like everyone's staring at me.
Masturbating in a cup feels very strange.
Masturbating in a cup will make a man change.

Oh I've done this before, but one thing's for sure.
I never had to stress about my aim.
With a cup it's a completely new game.
It doesn't really make me feel virile
When the room is so bland and yes sterile.
I do this to make sure that we can always have kids.
I just hope they never ask about what dear daddy did.
Masturbating in a cup feels very strange.
Masturbating in a cup will make a man change.

Oh I've done this before, but one thing's for sure.
I never had to stress about my aim
And I may never be the same.

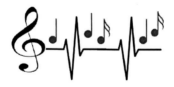

SONG 10

THE BATTLE

"Beating cancer is personal battle. It was one of the toughest opponents I have faced so far, and I think I did reasonably well. Touch wood."

~ Yuvraj Singh

"It doesn't take a hero to order men into battle. It takes a hero to be one of those men who goes into battle."

~ U.S. Army General Norman Schwarzkopf

"Some days there won't be a song in your heart. Sing anyway."

~ Emory Austin

A HEARTBEAT. I SAW the baby's heartbeat. It was amazing. I will be a daddy. Hey dad, I'm going to join you and become a dad." That was my journal entry on March 14, 2000, after I saw our first baby's heartbeat during an ultrasound. I still had a lot going through my head then, obviously, but I was totally thrilled by the heartbeat.

We didn't actually know yet if the child was "Klara" or "Henry" (or maybe Max), because we had decided to be surprised by our child's sex. We kept the name Klara in mind as it represents a blending of Allyson's middle name and her mom's name, plus, it's the Hungarian spelling (with a K for Klara) in homage to my heritage. The baby room we had created was great for either a boy or a girl.

We were also looking forward to our vacation in Greece and Istanbul in April. This overseas vacationing wasn't exactly annual for Allyson and me, but we would usually prefer November and Thanksgiving time to go somewhere new in Europe. The rates on travel and hotels were so much lower then. We'd both have a couple of free days off from work on Thanksgiving, Thursday and Friday, too, so that always helped us use fewer of our paid vacation days. This year, however, we had other plans for November: delivering our first child. So, April it was. We were planning this trip with our next-door neighbors. We'd been in this neighborhood for the past year and had become really good friends with them.

I was in pretty good physical shape at the time, but still questioning my health habits, wishing I would get more sleep and so on. I was struggling with work, too, in a different way, since I was still asking myself if I wanted to continue on there.

DRINK UP

On April 3, I was again at Emory Clinic — waiting once again to be poked and prodded. I was there for the standard post-op exam, complete with a CT scan and bloodwork. I was drinking the disgusting contrast medium for the scan. It was a chalky drink of barium sulfate, with the flavoring they add, which tastes a bit like Crystal Light. The medium is used to enhance the visibility of the gastrointestinal tract, and it is truly gross. I was trying to convince myself that the icky stuff tasted good enough to swallow three whole glasses of it. After chugging that down, I was ready for one CT scan. The nurse also inserted an IV with a big needle so that they could inject iodine for the second scan. I journaled that the nurse had white hair. He was very likable in my memory. I loved him for his skill and bedside manner. He was really good at inserting needles painlessly. I definitely appreciated that and his humor, too ("Don't worry — I haven't lost anyone yet. You're gonna feel like you wet your britches."). A second CT scan was taken after the iodine had finished coursing its way through me. I really remember that weird sensation of the medium going through my body. The sensation began in my head, and worked its way downward, creating a metallic taste in my mouth and concluded with... the feeling that I'd wet my britches. I just went with it all.

As I drank and waited, I journaled that I'd finished the music of "Life is Good" and I was looking forward to playing it for some people. Exams complete, I went back home, certainly feeling poked and jabbed, but none the worse for wear.

On April 6, I was in the doctor's office to get those exam results, and to ask about my continuing testicle pain. That was a strange, difficult, emotional day and I didn't journal for a couple of days as I was in a fog for a while.

On April 9, I journaled, "Wow, how things can change in just a few days." That was the day we were sitting on the plane to Greece to start our vacation week. I continued to journal, "Worst of all, they found a growth in my lung. I wasn't expecting this at all. Now I need another surgery." That had been the doctor's news on the sixth. That was the news that had made me feel so foggy and strange.

WATERMELON WARNING

The CT scan showed something that to me looked like a photo negative of a slice of watermelon with seeds. One of the seeds, which looked like a perfect isolated circle, was really a tumor. They were confident that this was a metastasis of the prior cancer, so they would be removing one third of that lung. After that, I would be transferred to an oncologist, who would most likely start me on chemo.

Interestingly, I don't remember any real discussion about alternatives. I do remember distinctly, in my haze, calling Allyson before leaving the clinic. At first, she thought I was joking when I said the cancer was back. She quickly realized it was no joke when I began sobbing, and immediately began changing her work travel plans so that she could come back home that night.

I was sent to speak directly to the thoracic surgeon that same day. He was a new cast member of my story.

As a side note, we met again over 10 years later. He told me that he never typically saw his patients again, except for a surgical follow-up. And there he was with his wife, a decade after my surgery, at my fund-raiser to raise money for a professional workshop of *Turning Thirty*. He was so taken with the show, and so pleased that I had reached out to him. He not only chatted with me, but made a $1,000 donation on the spot.

Anyway, after our return from Europe, I didn't journal again until April 30 — after the lung surgery and getting back at home to recover once again. I wrote, "Since I last wrote, I've been to Istanbul, I've had surgery, I'm in serious pain and on narcotics."

Not surprisingly, with a second procedure so close on the heels of the first one, I looked at it all as a battle. It's hard to pinpoint whether I penned this song before or after this lung surgery, but it is about surgery. All about the fight to eliminate cancer from my body through another surgery. In my journal, "Fight Song" was its working title. Later, once I started penning the words, it became "The Battle."

This song was designed to be a conversation between TC and the doctor. I envisioned it as a swordfight, actually, with mutual stabbing going on, as a metaphor for the surgical procedures I'd just had.

Weirdly for me, I am having TC say to the doctor, "No matter what you seem to do, I come back for him or perhaps you." I don't know why I needed to say this. I was compelled to not only write it, but retain it in the lyrics. At the time, it had only two meanings for me: that TC came back for me with new cancer, or he came back to give the doctor a new patient. It made me think that things weren't over yet for me. But many years after my own surgeries and remission, my urologist got prostate cancer himself. That is perhaps the story for another book (that he and I have actually discussed, as it happens). Cancer did come back for him later, in a third way I'd not thought of at the time.

The words demonstrate that I am thinking about this fight somewhat from the surgeon's standpoint, although the surgeon and I are facing it all together. The surgeon sings lines with TC. At the end of the song, TC stabs me and the doctor stabs TC.

It is modelled on the same theme as "Your Number's Up" and "We Will Face this Foe," but twice as slow — much more like a dirge. It is a death march, much more than a lively or upbeat march. It's definitely not a call to arms! The final music and words don't really resolve anything — just as after such a surgery, there is no resolution for a while. Again, this is a metaphor for the typical results of any surgical procedure.

"Because your number's up," says cancer, "it's time for you to sweat." And wait to see if this surgery will be the last one.

THE BATTLE

T.C.

We meet again.

DR. SAXON

Yes, it's true. Why do you keep doing what you do?

T.C.

Why do I? Why do we? You must grow tired of facing me.
No matter what you seem to do, I come back for him or perhaps you.

DR. SAXON

I don't care what you say. You won't win, not today.

T.C.

He was such an easy mark. I can keep you in the dark.

DR. SAXON

I must warn you. His will is strong.
Together we'll make sure you're gone.

T.C.
I grow tired of this senseless chatter.
Let's get to the heart of the matter.
Try to stop me or get out of my way.

DR. SAXON
Oh, we will stop you and you will pay.

T.C.
I will pay? Don't insult me.
I've made you pay already. Can't you see?
You know it's true.

DR. SAXON and CONLAN
We're strong. We're prepared.

T.C.
But are so afraid to see.

DR. SAXON and CONLAN
You will see.

T.C.
That your number's up.

DR. SAXON and CONLAN
Together.

T.C.
It's time for you to sweat.

DR. SAXON and CONLAN
The journey's led us here.

T.C.
Yes, your number's up.

DR. SAXON and CONLAN
Together.

T.C.
And thirty's all you get.

DR. SAXON and CONLAN
The end is very near.

T.C.
That's more than you deserved.

DR. SAXON and CONLAN
We must strike.

T.C.
I hate to wait so long.

DR. SAXON and CONLAN
Before long.

T.C.
Why should everything be so right?

DR. SAXON and CONLAN
If he thinks he'll win...

T.C.
Why should everything be so right?

DR. SAXON and CONLAN
If he thinks he'll win...

T.C.
When there is wrong?

DR. SAXON and CONLAN
He is wrong.

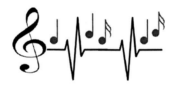

FOR A CHILD (TWO VERSIONS)

*"When my kids become wild and unruly, I use a nice safe playpen.
When they're finished, I climb out."*

~ Erma Bombeck

*"There really are places in the heart you don't even know exist —
until you love a child."*

~ Anne Lamott

*"I believe that what we become depends on what our fathers
teach us at odd moments, when they aren't trying to teach us.
We are formed by little scraps of wisdom."*

~ Umberto Eco, *Foucault's Pendulum*

O N MAY 22, 2000, I was about to get my first chemo treatment following the removal of one third of my lung. The chemo would last 12 weeks. I was reserved about it. I didn't want to get caught up kidding myself with any kind of prognosis. I was trying not to have hopes or expectations that might be dashed. The nurse walked me through the procedure and warned me about nausea and other practicalities, like avoiding greasy foods and such.

I wrote the lyrics of "For a Child 2" during this first infusion (or started it, at least) to keep my mind productively occupied.

I also journaled, "What a weird life. Testicular cancer. Metastasis. Baby. Musical." In addition to all the crazy stuff happening health-wise, it was also a bit action-packed at work. I went from a being a manager to getting a promotion to director around this time.

INSURANCE COVERAGE

We had both been signed up under Allyson's company benefits plan. She had unbelievable coverage (just a $100 deductible was all and all communications between providers and insurers were so easy). This eliminated the outrageous bills I had been getting before for care — some of which I didn't even expect. Her plan even covered our IVF process, which not all plans would have allowed. It was truly a crazy good insurance plan with Allyson's job. As for my own employer, the American Cancer Society, everyone was very, very good to me about my absences for doctor visits, surgery, chemo sessions, and recovery. Everyone was amazingly understanding.

SPERM BANK

Allyson's new pregnancy continued to go well. Parenthood was in the works. Even back in August, 1999, during my resistance to fatherhood, I knew that if anything happened to my ability to produce sperm, if I didn't have "reserves" and something went wrong as a result of the testicular cancer, I couldn't change my mind and have my own kids with Allyson. I couldn't count on continued sperm production. It was much too risky, given my type of cancer. Testicular cancer had moved us, as I said, to throw caution to the wind and have unprotected sex in August 1999. It was my first roll of the dice, because I just didn't know if/when I'd ever be all-in for fatherhood. I knew Allyson might get pregnant then, and I was willing to prepare for that, to be ready. My resistance sort of melted. I wanted to give us options for parenthood with my two visits to the sperm bank, and I guess, with the natural, unprotected sex, too.

Klara was conceived on a first IVF try — a pretty awesome result! Then Allyson stayed home for quite a while. By the time our second child Elliot's turn came, we were no longer benefitting from Allyson's generous insurance coverage, so we paid out of pocket for him (more like "out of house equity"). He was also conceived through IVF.

Our third child, Miles, was also a real roll of the dice. Allyson wanted more than our small family of four, as she comes from a 3-kid family. The risk? During a move to a new location, the lab lost my sperm. Panic! The clinic, however, came through for us. They decided to make up for this deeply distressing realization that we had no more shots at pregnancy — they did have the frozen embryos from when we had Elliot, but only them. With a Frozen Embryo Transfer (FET) process, we would have one shot left for pregnancy. Just one. We had no more sperm reserves and, after that FET, no more embryos. As luck had it, obviously, it worked. The FET was a success and, of course, our son Miles was a welcome, welcome addition. Allyson calls him our Bonus Miles. Interestingly, we decided on his name while looking at the quotes in The Artist's Way by Julie Cameron. I'll never forget it. The quote was "Do not fear mistakes — there are none," by Miles Davis.

CHANGING VIEWPOINTS

I journaled 'For a Child' with its shorter lyric in late October 1999. This is what we sing at the beginning of the musical, when my wife and I still do not agree about parenthood. I act resistant, totally unready. My wife is asking if I'd ever come around and make her a mother.

The longer "For a Child 2" is a much different song and sentiment, and its place is later in the show. I penned this lyric in May 2000, when my wife was already pregnant, and during the chemo following my lung surgery.

"For a Child 2" was constructed rather than just floating out. I wrote bits of it, then reversed the order they appear in and so on. It is based on the same theme as its first rendition. I'd consider it a slow ballad-type melody. The chords feel to me like a bit of magical wonder — inspiring, sort of reaching out to planets, like some of John Williams' Star Wars themes and that whole musical universe. Williams' work has always inspired me. That translated into the magical life of a new baby on its way.

This song is me coming to the sudden realization that, "Yeah, I like this idea. I'll be a Dad, just like my Dad. I love my Dad. He was a great Dad. Let's do this." I'm acting quite self-absorbed in the song — it's all about me. My mind is going wild for a child.

As I write lines, I try to interpret Allyson's typical reactions and thinking, so her character ends up just rolling her eyes and cracking some jokes. "Well, it is about time that idiot came around. He'd look good with four or five kids strapped to him."

And "Oh, thank God, he's finally lost the untimely error in his ways. Now I don't have to kill him!"

I change the key for each singer, both still in major keys, infusing that same magic and wonder of making a child, versus this down-to-earth topic of being parents. They end together in an uplifting, sort of majestic key.

I'm really proud of the close of this song. It's so satisfying to me. It's just really pretty back-and-forth melodies and resolution. I even actually found three rhymes to 'child' — I was really happy with this song!

FOR A CHILD

CONLAN

For a child, I am not ready for a child. I have great fear

For a child makes me wonder if to her I'll be less dear.

I'm not wild about the thought of changing everything around me,

For a child might change the person she will be.

HALLE

For a child, I wish he'd understand. For a child is what I long.

It frightens me that he might see the time as always wrong.

I'm not wild about the thought of never having a family,

For without a child I'm afraid of the person I might be.

FOR A CHILD 2
CONLAN
For a child I am now ready.

For a child I understand
Why she would plea so much to me.
The time is now at hand.
It surprises me that there could be a new outlook in me
For a child won't change the people we will be.

HALLE

For a child it's about time
That that bastard's come around.
I thought I'd have to withhold sex
Until good sense was found.
Oh, thank god he finally lost the untimely error in his ways.
*For if not more careful he'd darn well discover the end of
his days.*

CONLAN

For a child I'd be a father.
The mere thought could drive one mad.
I can scarcely fathom what 'twill be to be a dad.
Maybe only now I see what it is that I could be.

HALLE

Look at him. What a shock. On and on he goes,
Once again lost in himself, where that is god only knows.

CONLAN and HALLE

For a child we are now ready.

CONLAN/HALLE

For a child I understand
And the time is now at hand.

CONLAN

It's such a gift!

HALLE

One I've always planned...

CONLAN

All my doubts I've reconciled

HALLE

For upon us he has smiled.

CONLAN and HALLE

Now we are both wild, for a child.

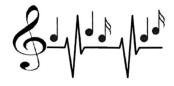

HAVE A BALL

"I don't think it's possible to have a sense of tragedy without having a sense of humor."

~ Christopher Hitchens

"The only way to make sense out of change is to plunge into it, move with it, and join the dance."

~ Alan Watts

"One person's craziness is another person's reality."

~ Tim Burton

IF IT SOUNDS, FROM earlier songs, as though many of the songs I wrote for the musical came to me fairly quickly (and they did), it will become clear that the next few took form over quite a longer period. In fact, I worked on the remaining songs off and on from about May through November 2000. I wove back and forth among these next songs as my creativity for them — and my physical stamina — allowed.

A lot was going on in my life in those months, with much, but not all of it, about the cancer.

DOWN BUT NOT OUT

On May 24, 2000, I wrote, "Down with cisplatin." Cisplatin is a chemotherapy drug, credited with turning around testicular cancer to be treatable, and one of the three drugs (bleomycin, etoposide, and cisplatin — "BEP") I was taking. It was nasty. You are literally being given platinum. I wrote, "I hope I control the nausea. This is not cool. I get cold when I'm getting infused and these infusions are somehow making me physically heavier."

In response to my question about why I kept getting heavier, my oncologist said, "You're on steroids, that's why you feel heavier."

"So how come I don't look like Ahnold?"

"You're on the type of steroids that give you a nice *pear* shape."

Well, day after day, I actually did gain weight. One time, in just 3 days I'd gained maybe five pounds.

I was feeling really rotten as a result of the chemo infusions. Yes, I was gaining weight, but not from overeating. Food didn't taste good. Eating had gotten tricky. Things tasted strange or unappetizing and I didn't feel good after eating. I would get random cravings. For instance, I hadn't had a bologna sandwich since I was a kid and I craved one. That was funny. But we went with it. Anything to get food in me.

We went out and got the makings for one, and let me say that it tasted awesome!

THE FAMILY DRUGGIE

I had a shoebox filled with close to 30 prescription medicines by the end of my chemo — meds to counter side effects of the chemo, new meds to counteract side effects of those first meds. Crazy! To poison the cancer, I poisoned myself.

In addition to all these prescriptions during chemo, I also had kind friends get me marijuana. I talked about it with my oncologist, who said it was up to me whether to try it or not, but suggested that I do not smoke it, since bleomycin can affect your lungs. So we researched online how to cook with it, and it was far and away the most effective at managing the nausea and other symptoms of chemo. Allyson said the difference was night and day — with all the other anti-emetics, including Marinol (synthetic marijuana), I still suffered. With marijuana, she says, I practically became myself again. I agree. I am heartened by the growing legal acceptance of this drug for medical use.

I didn't journal much in June. On July 8, I wrote, "I've just listened to 'For a Child 2' that I had finally recorded." I also journaled that I was having strong visions of my late father.

On August 7, I journaled, "I don't feel great, but I had my reawakening this morning. I cried. For the first time since March, I cried. I actually feel the end is near — I see a vision of a highway under construction with a sign saying 'Construction Ends.'" I was seeing light at the end of this cancer eradication tunnel, the end of chemo, the end of this "cancer detour" on my road. Somehow, I started thinking I was going to make it.

I was taking Benadryl and giving myself shots. I had taken a liking to cinnamon gum and its "vain attempt at intensity."

August 15, as the last entry that day in my journal, I wrote (I presume with some relief), "I'm done. I'm done. I'm done.

No more chemo. Time to watch (to see if anything comes back)." On September 18, my chest port — a long-term way of delivering the chemo infusions I had been getting — was removed. That was a bit unnerving, a little spooky.

LONG BEAUTIFUL HAIR

I was closing in on October and my hair was starting to grow back. I'd lost it all after the first round of chemo, around the third week. I touched my head one day, and came away with a handful of hair. I was pulling it out easily by hand (no pain or pulling involved, by the way — it was all simply loose by then), so we went straight to the hair salon. As an attempt perhaps at macabre humor, I grabbed and pulled out a piece of my hair right in front of the hairdresser through her shop window, and she waved me into the chair and gave me a buzz cut. "Emergency, no appointment required."

It is a little-known fact that *all* body hair goes, not just the hair on your head. Ear hair, eyebrows, eyelashes, nose hair, all the cilia of the throat, and so on. Nasty effect. I only realized what function hair fulfilled when I didn't have any.

Over this whole spring, summer, and fall period, I was asking myself whether thirteen songs for the musical would be enough. "Have a Ball" came together. It was completed as the third of the four songs that came to me in this period. In my journal, I wrote about the song concept, "I'd like to write a song with double entendre that refers both to losing one testicle and to having fun." Losing a testicle and poking fun at it by having a ball. Finally. I'm not sure I could've written this humorous a song a year earlier, given the emotional turmoil of cancer at that time.

The "Have a Ball" words started coming to me on July 9, when I started to journal loads of potential thoughts and words for it that never made it to the final version. Some of the concepts I journaled for this music included, "Jump, jive, and wail—swing, boogie!" I loved working on and writing these songs—this is what I craved and loved doing then. By October 1, I hadn't finished this song and I journaled, "I need to get creative for these last two songs." Time to finish the lyrics for "Have a Ball."

Conlan sings this song with three men. "Have a Ball" is a swing tune with two-part harmonies for the clown-like doctors. I knew I wanted to poke at the removed testicle—in the show, the music stops and the testicle bounces across the stage with the doctors chasing after it. As in "Your Number's Up," the doctors are up to their crazy antics.

This is a very upbeat swing tune, communicating the song's basic emotion of gaiety and laughter, but it is offset by the lyrics expressing the seriousness of losing a testicle to cancer. It's not an easy choice. It's scary. You feel solitary when you are face-to-face with the decision to have a ball removed. I used to be tough—I used to have balls. I used to think they'd always be around. Now I only have a ball. And this song.

HAVE A BALL

I used to think they'd always be around.

No reason to think otherwise, I'd found.

Then one day everything had changed

And my thoughts on the subject were completely rearranged.

It occurred to me that something had gone wrong

And I'd have to act to fix it before long.

I had little time I had to make the call,

So I thought, 'Why should I worry when I can just have a ball?'

Have a ball, have a ball! Oh, I'm up against a wall.

If I let them have a ball, there's only one left. Yes, that's all.
They say I need just one. They say it won't hurt at all.
Well, if that's what it takes, then baby have a ball.
Now you might think that it's an easy choice
And you would not be afraid to raise your voice,
But let me tell you it's not simple at all, no,
When you're face to face with the decision to have a ball.
Have a ball, have a ball. Oh, I'm up against a wall.
If I let them have a ball, there's only one left. Yes, that's all.
They say I need just one. They say it won't hurt at all.
Well, if that's what it takes, then baby have a ball.
Oh, it's scary. Yes, it's very solitary, makes me wary
Like an unnecessary adversary. It seems so involuntary.
Why am I the only guy whose happy life's gone so awry?
I used to be tough. I used to stand tall.
I used to have balls, but now I only have a ball.
Have a ball, have a ball. Oh, I'm up against a wall.
If I let them have a ball, there's only one left. Yes, that's all.
They say I need just one. They say it won't hurt at all.
Well, if that's what it takes, though it gives me the shakes,
Please don't make any mistakes and baby have a ball.

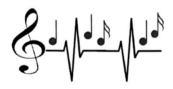

SOMETIMES

"If there is no struggle, there is no progress."

~ Frederick Douglass

"It's got to do with putting yourself in other people's shoes and seeing how far you can come to truly understand them."

~ Christian Bale

THROUGH MOST OF THIS period, I had been having angst on and off about work. I got my promotion at work, only to be out on chemo days. I had to stay home on those days for the most part, since I was wrung out. And all the while, I did what I could to stay connected with work. It was hard.

Allyson and I were nesting, building the room for our first baby. We painted it light blue. We were coming up to the due date for our first child in November 2000. We were both so excited — me, too, despite being wrung like a rag so much of the time.

The name of the paint was Santorini Blue — coincidentally, Santorini was where we went in April for our Greece vacation. My travel neighbor, in addition to being a world-class horn player, was an amazing wood worker and helped with some permanent wall drawers and such later in that project. I made a drawing so that we could arrange furniture. I also finished work on the porch of the house. I was trying to keep active and busy with home projects in spite of it all.

Music was still part of what I did with my time, of course. I bought a Kurzweil keyboard and started recording with that. I'd used my old recording equipment long enough. I met Kurzweil at an event sometime after my purchase. He's known as a kind of futurist, having invented optical character recognition and other things. You can Google him, if you are not familiar with his work. Interestingly, Raymond Kurzweil would actually come into my life again years later.

DÉJÀ VU

My wife and I were at Mount Washington Resort in New Hampshire for another of Allyson's company retreats on July 28. "Here we are again," I thought, one year later. Last year at her retreat was where I discovered the lump in my testicle. We travelled to the retreat between chemo sessions — at that time, it was the only way I could go anywhere. "I can't wait to be done with chemo," I thought. It was like a mantra.

It was about 2 weeks, no more, after finishing the 12 to 13 weeks of chemo. Before chemo began, I was sure I could handle it. I was strong. I could do it easily. Wrong. It had totally wrung me out. Sometimes I was just plain passed out in bed. And some side effects felt completely out of my control, like my white blood cell count, which no amount of attitude seemed to improve.

ALLYSON'S SONG

I was really nauseous a lot of the time. My wife was still working and trying to juggle pregnancy and her work with waiting on me. And one night when I was totally out of it, unbeknownst to me, she broke down from the weight of it all. She sat on our front stoop after dark, and just cried and cried. A neighbor saw her — I was out of the picture, virtually unconscious — and he came over, quietly sat with her and helped her cry.

That image, which I hadn't even witnessed, drove what I wanted to say for this song. Reflecting on this experience of hers after it was reported to me, I asked myself, "What would she have said that day?" I heard her in my head, saying, "What about me? I can't stand to see him this way. What on earth am I supposed to do?" This introspection took me out of myself and into my beloved wife's emotions and thoughts.

I had not yet focused a song on Allyson and her journey through my cancer. It had been all about me and my cancer — just TC and me.

I will always think of this as Allyson's song. She was my love and my inspiration, and I wrote the words as I felt she might have been experiencing my cancer.

She still says it is one of the hardest songs of the musical for her to listen to.

On July 9, Allyson's song had me journaling the words that would become the song lyrics. I wrote the words in paragraph form, and then broke it up into rhyming lines. I completed it on August 27. It was fairly easy for me to do a stream of consciousness of the words and I retained much of that first inspiration in the final lyrics. The song had tentative titles of "Killing Me, Too" and "Allyson's Song." It was when I made stanzas that I wrote the final title, "Sometimes."

This song jumps around in time signature, although it is mostly a 3/4 waltz feeling. It is similar to "How Could This Be?" in that regard, with an extra beat slid in, or moving back to 4/4-time in the middle. Conlan went through feelings in "How Could This Be?" and this is Halle's version — Halle's story, her own feelings, and what she is going through.

The song is mostly in a minor key, when Halle is thinking, "This isn't the way it was supposed to be." When she becomes nostalgic, imagining how her life might be, the song goes to a major key in 4/4-time. When time signatures change, it is to express Halle's emotions of sorrow, as she is wondering, "What if it gets worse?" A 3/4 waltz in a minor key is her sadness and grief.

SOMETIMES

Sometimes I stand.

Sometimes I fall.

Sometimes I wonder if anyone understands at all.

What about me?

Why did this even have to happen at all?

I don't care about some baby. I care about him.

I don't want to be alone should he fall.

Sometimes I feel like we will be fine.

We're lucky. We'll get through it and we'll be okay.

This is just a minor detour...

But sometimes it doesn't feel that way.

What if it doesn't get better? What if it gets worse?

What if we battle this for years until it finally breaks him and me?

It's such an unknown and I want to know.

I want it to be known and I want it to be good.

This is not how my life is supposed to be.

I'd have a husband who loves me and treats me so well.

We'd have carloads of children with stories to tell,

Learning and growing and caring,

Yearning and going and sharing.

This is the way it was meant for me,

Not the way it has turned out to be.

I can't stand to see him this way,

Tired and pained and suffering all day.

I think of what might be and don't know what to do.

I don't want to live if he's not here too.

The worst part is the man I can turn to, can lean on, who keeps me sane

Is the one who can't help me, the one who's in pain.

Dear god, what on earth am I supposed to do?

This horrible nightmare is killing me too.

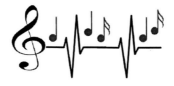

SONG 14

POISON

"Chemotherapy tests your sanity."

~ Melissa Etheridge

"All things are poisons, for there is nothing without poisonous qualities. It is only the dose which makes a thing poison."

~ Paracelsus

"I just wanted them to die," said Poison.
"They didn't have to make such a drama about it."

~ Chris Wooding, 'Poison'

SENSORY DEPRIVATIONS

A S A CONSEQUENCE OF the chemo, my five senses were off, and that is an understatement. My sense of touch, sight, and so on were all affected in some way. My eyeglasses didn't give me the same sharp focus during chemo as pre-chemo, for instance.

I journaled, "I hope I get my voice and hearing back." The distortion of my hearing affected how I heard my own voice from inside my head. My singing ability seemed off on the high notes, weaker, harder to control, a little scratchy. Kind of like a bad sore throat when we have a cold. We are so close to our voices — we hear ourselves in our heads, but my family and others never really commented (if they noticed at all).

My audio frequency range was reduced — lower highs and lows, but higher mid-range frequencies that seemed distorted. Mixing songs I'd recorded was a challenge because I was not hearing what I was doing well enough.

Yes, my voice has gotten better over the years since then, but, as I write this nearly two decades later, I don't think my hearing ever fully recovered.

On October 13, I saw the oncologist for a check-up. No CT scans. He didn't know the answer when I asked about getting my voice and hearing back again — no one had asked him that before! I guess the musician and audiophile in me noticed it, whereas others wouldn't. But by going online, I found people who corroborated my experience of messed-up sensory capability. I saw with a tiny bit of relief that I wasn't alone.

That same day, I wrote, "I'm in a bit of angst about work." I was still trying to figure this aspect of my life out. I was back at work, feeling like I was still sort of struggling, though, with the idea that I should be doing something different. No answers were within my reach yet.

SHOWTIME

On October 16, 2000, I journaled about my wish to do a live one-person version of this complete show. Just to try it out on a friendly audience. I do like all the songs, but that never means they will all be well-received by others. A test run might be in order, I thought. However, I had not scripted all of the dialog yet. That would take almost another year.

In August 2001, I sent the music to some theaters in Atlanta — and one of the theaters asked me to send the script as well. It wasn't ready then, either! I solicited Jonathan's help (a good friend from childhood who was doing an MFA degree in theater at the time) and he responded, "Sounds like fun!" We discussed preparing both a single-person script and a full cast script. He worked from my rough draft. The musical book (perhaps better known as a libretto, the text for a musical theater production) was happily underway with friendly help from Jonathan. Nothing like a theater showing interest to put the fire under you!

"Poison" is one of the three songs I composed over much of 2000, as I mentioned earlier. This one is more or less the third of the three. The stream of consciousness on this song came and went over time, slowly turning into lyric format. In my third round of writing, I finished this song. "Poison" was complete by mid-October.

For this lyric, I was influenced by my choice of having made testicular cancer (TC) a personified character of the story. Chemo and my experience of preparation for each infusion, the bags of infusions themselves, losing my sensory capacity, losing my hair — all this colored my view of this "poison" used against TC. I have to say it: I felt that a part of me was dying. Thus, the word "poison" seemed right. It was foremost in my mind that we are poisoning the host.

BLACK MAGIC

The concept of doctor-turned-wizard was strong — as was "black magic" — with some suggestion of an eerie, weird thing happening in the background of my awareness. "A tumor is a rumor, cancer is the answer, chemo is the cure" was a medical school rhyme I heard from a doctor that gave me the idea of infusions as magic potions. Chemo was basically me going to a wizard for the magic, curative potion I needed.

I once set eyes on my personal medical file. It was, at that point, a giant printed folder. Remember, this was before electronic health records became prevalent. The file was started with my cancer diagnosis a year earlier. I sat and looked for a moment through my own records. The urologist couldn't help me anymore — I understood this. His phase of care was over. He knew someone who could continue my care, though, and off I went to the oncologist to let him add to that mountain of a file. The oncologist was the right person now to make the cancer disappear without another trace.

In spite of jotting down random ideas and stream of conscious thoughts since springtime, it was from August to October that these three songs really got my fullest attention. On October 1, I journaled some word associations for the concept of poison. Sleight of hand, magician, Jedi, mystery, wizard and so on were part of the list.

The music for these scary words has an almost orchestral flavor. For the wizard's opening words, it is grandiose like a piano concerto backed by the big string section and wind instruments.

In the second part of the song, my character sings about what it is like to receive this magic potion, and there are eerie, creepy, and lush chords to support the creepiness of my feelings and the scariness of the chemo experience for any patient. The vocal arrangement calls for falsetto from my character in order to better depict my increasing weakness from the treatments. Then the wizard comes back at the end, singing back and forth with me, and closes the song with a full voice. The wizard knows TC is really much, much worse off than I am.

To this day, my brother cannot easily listen to this song. It makes his skin crawl. He can't imagine how anyone could go through a treatment like this. I hear you, brother. I wonder, too.

I am particularly tickled by my success at inserting the word "assuage." As a kid, the Todd Rundgren song called "Honest Work" used the word and it came back to me:

I know I'm not the only one

To fall beneath the wheel

Such company cannot assuage

The loneliness I feel.

It was fun to sneak that word in…

POISON

WIZARD

I've analyzed your enemy. I know just what he needs.

He can't exist without you. It's off of you he feeds,

So if you want him off your back, you've come to the right place.

I can help you make him go away, disappear without a trace,

So settle down, relax. No cause for a commotion.

I know the secret formula. I have the magic potion.

I'll share with you the answer to make this one a ghost

To kill this parasite
We must poison the host.

CONLAN (*getting infusions*)

A part of me is dying,
I can feel it fade away.
Why must this be so trying?

WIZARD

I don't know what to say.

CONLAN

The sky has become overcast.
The sea's no longer grand.
The air is all polluted.
The soil has turned to sand.
I must be in a nightmare.
Please tell me it's not real.
Nothing could hope to assuage
How horrible I feel.
When will this be over?

WIZARD

You need to drink some more.

CONLAN
I could not take another sip.

WIZARD
That's only one of four.
I know that you must suffer.
Don't worry, troubled friend.
Though it may feel like an eternity,
Soon all of this will end,
So drink up all your poison
And sleep the whole night through,
For when the nightmare's over
He will be worse off than you.

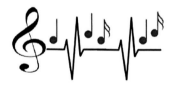

NOT DONE YET

*"I never see what has been done;
I only see what remains to be done."*

~ Attributed to the Buddha

*"So, what is my story? I don't know.
It's long and twisted and not quite finished yet."*

~ Caitlyn Paige

*"Existence is a series of footnotes to a vast,
obscure, unfinished masterpiece."*

~ Vladimir Nabokov

A S I TRIED TO complete "Poison," I had an inkling that the story needed more. I knew it wasn't the last song I would want to pen for the whole story to be told. "Not Done Yet" (for which I had penned that exact title way back when the idea for a musical came to me) is the song that makes it a wrap.

In the context of the musical production, it would be fitting, I thought, to have TC — Testicular Cancer — rise again. "You thought you killed me, but I'm not done yet." That is the origin of this last song and its name.

I do remember that I imagined that I was done with cancer after the RPLND. Another reason to write "Not Done Yet" was the memory of the fear I had when it was again detected in my lung. I was crushed when it returned. I think anyone with a cancer experience has this fear to some degree, right alongside the courage to live life in full remission.

CANCERVERSARY

In our home, we have a little decorative, old-fashioned chalkboard. We used to jot our To Do list on it. Back then, in the year 2000, right along with Basement/Yard Sale, Become Mommy and Daddy, and Repot Plants was ... *CURE CANCER.* To this day, that last entry remains on the board.

Upon successful completion of chemo, I imagined and talked about a 10-year Cancerversary. I never have held such a celebration. I guess it was a superstitious thing, like too much arrogant thinking about having seen the last of the cancer will invite it back. I could almost hear TC laughingly snicker in the background that he was "Not done yet. Not done." My healthy respect for its potential to come back has kept me from any celebration — except for our celebration of life through parenthood with Allyson.

Despite my life purpose crisis in relation to my work at the ACS during my cancer era, I spent over 20 years there. I believe that some of that crisis in 1999 and 2000 was that I was simply dealing with a terrifying personal dilemma at the same time that my management was attempting to make some significant changes in my department. My cancer happened during a major department downsizing and reorganization. Intellectually, I got that it was a fairly typical strategy for large and established corporations to go through periodically. I had never yet in my career experienced such change. I still experienced lots of angst personally. There was also lots of angst amongst my co-workers about their job security. The downsizing was severe, reducing the department size by almost 75%. Fortunately, it was handled very well. But the place and space I was in personally gave me a difficult disconnect to manage in myself. I couldn't have done a huge Spring Cleaning in my own home in those months, let alone in my job! I am, in hindsight, glad someone else was in charge of that phase of development of the company. A different person came to be in charge of the department after this shift. I was happy to stay with the corporation and work under his direction. I let go of my angst right along with finding my strength and health again.

This song has a double-edged title. I was not done with the musical story and this wrapped it. I remembered that at every stage of my treatments and tests I had the hope that I was done. Letting go of the surgical past, I would think, "I am moving on." Not yet. I'm getting the feeling I'm not done yet. TC's story, I fear, is not quite finished. The fear is lurking — TC may rise again.

This song is very minimalist. TC sings. A high register piano accompanies it. I put key changes, from A minor to B flat major and back, in such a brief song. I wanted it to feel a little creepy, with the sense that something a bit invisible, yet fairly dramatic, was happening in the background. The final chord does not resolve, just as cancer does not. Both leave you hanging. As though you will never quite be done with it...

NOT DONE YET

They think that I'm defeated.

I'm so misunderstood.

They think the blade had slain me.

They think I'm gone for good.

But I'm not done yet. Don't underestimate me.

Yes, I'll be back. Just you wait and see.

No, I'm not done yet. I'm just keeping out of sight.

Don't think that this is over for I've just begun to fight.

LESSONS LEARNED

"Tell me and I forget. Teach me and I remember.
Involve me and I learn."

~ Benjamin Franklin

IF YOU ARE LIKE me, there are many Ah-Ha! moments of realization and learning during, as well as long after, the journey of healing yourself from cancer. Here are some of my lessons learned. I hope they are beneficial to you, too.

1. Enjoy every good and bad moment, because now — this very moment — is all you ever have. Our lives are just a succession of right nows, one after the other. Focus on this moment. I found that all the others will take care of themselves.

2. Soul search. What do you enjoy? What and who is important to you? Be honest with yourself and your loved ones.

3. Listen to your intuition. Whatever you call it, intuition is that wisdom that comes from God, your Highest Consciousness, angels, your life experience, and guides. Act on it.

4. Discover *The Artist's Way* by Julia Cameron. Along with the actual composition of what became the musical, journaling as defined by Ms. Cameron

kept me going in positive ways. Adapt something like this to your days ... and nights.

5. After your soul search (which, granted, may unfold over quite a long time), take actions to maximize the time you spend doing what you love and with the people you love.

- Become stingier with your time. When you lose yourself, keep doing that. If it feels wrong, it probably is, so stop doing that.

- Reduce the number of things you dislike, but must do. Your case might be that you hate to clean house and to reduce that, you hire someone to come in and do it. Or simplify/fix the things you don't enjoy, but must do. One case for me of this was installing a laundry chute serving all floors of my home, so that I would no longer have to "do the stairs" with armloads of smelly laundry. It was a convenience for us all in the end, but the change was motivated by me fixing something I disliked. Figure out how to make even the tedious tasks in your daily routine enjoyable.

- I see humor being about balance in my life. We are not just drama, trauma, and tears. We balance it out with laughter and humor and joking. There's something funny about everything, and if we look, we can usually find it — even in our darkest hours. For example, one of the ways Allyson and I found to cope during that time was to greatly speed up what's known as the five stages of grief — denial, anger, bargaining, depression and acceptance. Whenever we got troubling news, we would quickly make faces representing each stage. It was our humorous attempt to get it over with and move on. It actually helped. It's usually only a matter of shifting your perspective just a tad. It's there.

- Don't wait — it usually takes adversity to bring about a turning point in one's life. Seize the opportunity to get your life (and your attitude) the way you want it as you heal your body. Let go of painful or non-supportive relationships. Let go of a job that never suited you. There are other people and more jobs out there. Clean it all up.

- Don't just say it, do it. This supports the prior advice, really. If intuition gives you something, don't just notice it. Act on it. That way, in my experience, we get more and more beneficial help from "on high."

- Money is only good when it buys experiences and freedom. Have real goals to travel, spend more time with family, own a house, etc.

- Finally, gratitude. Be grateful for those who are in your life and support you through thick and thin. Get in the habit of gently but confidently saying, "I appreciate you" to those who lend a hand in any way. Those who say, "If you need anything just let me know" may never come back, but those who actually cook for you in their home and bring over dinner? Man, they surely are keepers! Express your thanks. You are really and truly blessed.

NEW PERSPECTIVES

*"Each day, as you get older, there is a new
perspective on life. It's a progression of some sort."*

~ John Hurt

*"When you do find humor in trying times, one of
the first and most important changes you experience
is that you see your perplexing problems in a new
way — you suddenly have a new perspective on
them."*

~ Allen Klein

I have been down a path that changed my life. No longer do I look at things the same way.

I now have a healthy respect for every follow-up visit to the doctor. I have a new view on the medical profession and all the years and years each specialist spends to become a life-saving angel.

The hardest moments in my life now seem to pale in comparison to the time when I was fighting to stay alive, using knives and poison. I now have three beautiful, healthy (and I hope happy) children — Klara, Elliot, and Miles.

I realize that every single living, breathing moment is one to be savored. It doesn't matter whether it is easy or difficult, good or bad, right or wrong. I don't know what the end of this story will be. I just hope it comes many, many years from now.

MY CREW

I WAS FORTUNATE TO be surrounded by so many loving people through my illness, the development of my musical, all the way to the writing of this book. Though I could write another book just to thank everyone who helped me, I would like to thank:

Allyson Willner – My soulmate, best friend, and life partner who also graciously agreed to be my wife. Her continued tolerance of me and my general craziness is a source of both amazement and unending love and appreciation.

Klara, Elliot, and Miles – Our three miracle children who each continue to amaze me as the years go by. If you had any doubts, I hope the story I tell in this book helps you understand who I was during my illness and how that experience, along with fatherhood, has made me who I am today.

My Family – Mom and Dad, who I can't thank enough for all they've done for me — I miss them both dearly; my brother, John Willner, who has been my hero for as long as I can remember; and my sister JoAnne Molnar, who is a fellow cancer survivor, and I *like* her (she'll laugh!).

Allyson's Family – Karen and Tom Lacey, and Craig and Todd Bower, who are all as dear to me as my own parents and siblings; Allison Bower and Melissa Bower, my fellow out-laws! Bruce Bower, whose generosity and spirit never cease to amaze me; and Diana O'Neill, whose unending kindness helped inspire me to write the song "I'm Here for You."

Jonathan Uffelman – My wonderful, talented, and lifelong friend who shared his creativity and writing skills to help me write the scenes and dialog for my musical.

Andrew Blais – Another wonderful, talented, and lifelong friend (Andy, Jonathan, and I were known as the *Triumvirate*) who was a ridiculously good friend through my cancer experience and to this day.

Ben Wakeman – My amazing friend, talented musician and writer, who was there with me through my journey, and even wrote about it in one of his songs, "Half In Shadow Half In Light."

> *When you surrendered to the force that you call fate*
>
> *You cut the tether and began to float away*
>
> *I gave you up for dead before you returned for good*
>
> *Smiling like a man who'd seen the other side and lived to tell*

Everyone who helped make a staged show of Turning Thirty, The Musical – My dear friends the Duncans: Bill Duncan, a fellow cancer survivor and theater professional whose skills made the show and the workshop possible, and the talented and lovely Pam Duncan who performed so brilliantly as TC that she reprised the role in every performance I've done; Adam Coletta, my brother from another mother and super talented musician who performed all of the guitars at every performance; Lee Hansen, who continues to lend his talents to performances even now for Center Stage Education; and Kristi Budd, Jose Cordero, Stan Joseph, Talmadge Hickman, and Lee Nunn, all terrific friends who sing, act, and play in the show.

The talented professionals in the workshop of my show – Michael Fauss, Scott Warren, Jeremy Wood, Laura Floyd, Jeremy Varner, Bryan Mercer, Pam Duncan, Carlos Rivera,

Luke Weathington, Stan Joseph, Adam Coletta, and all the supporters of the workshop who made it possible.

Anne McSweeney – My partner-in-crime who combined forces with me to change healthcare education, and who helped find an exciting new avenue where my show can help people and make a difference. She is indeed the yin to my yang.

Those who made this book a reality – David Harris, who planted the seed and encouraged me to write this book; Tamma Ford, who helped me through the whole creative process and whose professionalism, patience, and experience was a true blessing; Benard Owuondo, who helped me get this book from draft to nearly finished product; Louis Leon, for his photography expertise and efforts to capture just the right images; and Emily Pualwan, whose publishing and marketing expertise as well as infectious enthusiasm helped get this book to the finish line and beyond.

Finally, to all the healthcare professionals who helped me survive cancer: Dr. Issa, my urologist, good friend, and the model for Dr. Saxon; Dr. Tahn, my oncologist; Dr. Manseur, my thoracic surgeon and huge supporter of the show; and of course all the angels — my nurses, administrative staff, and fertility clinic personnel who were there through it all: diagnosis, surgeries, chemotherapy, healing, and creating my family.

WHEN I DID THE professional workshop of my musical, one of the actors told me how helpful it would be for those in the medical community to see the show. He felt that there was an audience who would not only enjoy the show on its own merits, but who would truly learn something valuable to them and their work about the patient experience.

Fast forward a few years to that fateful phone call from Anne McSweeney. Anne created a company called CEU Creations to make continuing education courses for healthcare workers that were not your same old, boring classes. She read about my musical in a newspaper article and reached out to see if we could combine efforts.

Today, we have Center Stage Education, a company designed to deliver keynote presentations and CE classes for healthcare professionals using music. Of course, our first and signature event is to teach about the patient experience using Turning Thirty, The Musical.

You can find out more about our work at www.centerstageeducation.com.